MANAGING BOUNDARIES
IN THE
HEALTH PROFESSIONS

MANAGING BOUNDARIES IN THE HEALTH PROFESSIONS

JOHN G. BRUHN
New Mexico State University
Las Cruces, New Mexico

and

HAROLD GRUMET LEVINE
and
PAULA L. LEVINE
University of Texas Medical Branch at Galveston
Galveston, Texas

With a New Introduction by the Authors

PERCHERON PRESS
A Division of Eliot Werner Publications, Inc.
Clinton Corners, New York

Library of Congress Control Number 2002101607

This Percheron Press paperback edition of *Managing Boundaries in the Health Professions* is an unabridged republication of the edition published by Charles C. Thomas in 1993 supplemented with a new introduction by the authors.

ISBN 0-9712427-7-1

Copyright © 2002 Percheron Press
A Division of Eliot Werner Publications, Inc.
PO Box 268, Clinton Corners, New York 12514
http://www.eliotwerner.com

Printed in the United States of America

Dedicated To
STEWART WOLF, M.D. and WILLIAM W. SCHOTTSTAEDT, M.D.
Administrators in Health Science Centers who inspired loyalty, modeled excellence, and created a working environment that challenged individuals to expand their horizons.

INTRODUCTION TO THE
PERCHERON PRESS EDITION

Boundaries set limits, restrict access, and thus control behavior. There have always been ways of controlling behavior in health care through accessibility, availability, and affordability. With managed care these methods have become more bureaucratized and rigid. Before managed care people could choose and access both primary care providers and specialists with relative ease. As public policymakers became concerned with the rising costs of health care, especially specialty care, cost controls were initiated. As the government and insurance companies have managed health care costs, they have also gained greater control over who can have access to certain providers and their services. In addition, the funders of health care have influenced how health providers practice their professions. For example, physicians and patients are forced to relate to each other in a narrower range and more of physicians' actions are being dictated and standardized (Bruhn 2001a). The problems and issues discussed by physicians and patients are largely limited by what is reimbursable.

Rigid boundaries help to control financial costs but many social inequities related to health status and health care have not changed as a result of managed care. Our society's approach to health care is still multitiered; a minimum level of services is available to patients in the lowest tier. Depending on one's ability to pay, a person can receive the best health care in the world or not fare as well as one's contemporaries in Europe (Lewis and Parent 2001). National health care costs (projected to reach 16.2 percent of the Gross Domestic Product by 2008) continue to rise despite managed care. More than 40 million Americans have no health insurance. Uninsured citizens are usually financially poor; subsistence needs preempt those of health even when there are severe symptoms. Health care is usually a catastrophic event. Managed care is not concerned with citizens' health status until they enter the system for care. Thus any concerns about prevention and health education to increase the responsibility for—and responsiveness to—one's own health are minimal or nonexistent.

vii

Managed care encourages a fragmented approach to health care. A patient becomes a series of problems, some of which are reimbursable but others not; the interrelationship of these problems, especially as they relate to the total functioning of patients and their quality of life, is not a high priority of managed care or the health providers who must be concerned with diagnosing and treating reimbursable conditions.

Rigid boundaries keep people apart and are not conducive to building partnerships or teams. More than one-half of the households in the United States changed physicians during the past two years chiefly because people were not happy with their physicians. HMO representatives advise clients to select a primary care physician from a list of participating providers about whom the client knows little. The HMO encourages clients to visit their chosen physician prior to an emergency, advising clients that they can change physicians up to eight times a year if they are not satisfied. Such a message conveys to clients that the physician-patient relationship is not expected to last long enough to establish trust, only long enough to see if the patient likes the physician as a person and gets what he or she wants.

Primary care physicians in HMOs refer to specialists, but frequently the primary care physician and the specialist do not communicate; hence the patient often assumes responsibility for informing the primary care provider about the results of the tests that the specialist conducted. Often when patients change HMOs and primary care physicians, their medical records are not transferred and they must chronicle the details of their medical history each time they change physicians. While greater responsibility and autonomy for one's health care can be advantageous, it is not uncommon for patients (especially the elderly) to feel overwhelmed by the bureaucracy of boundaries.

Brokers and Boundary Spanners

The traditional health professional-patient dyad has evolved into a triad of payer-health professional-patient. The payer is the dominant decision maker; the health professional is the broker of services; the patient is the consumer. The basic tenet of this relationship is negotiation. For example, a physician makes a diagnosis and formulates an approach to treatment. The physician and patient discuss the treatment options that the payer will cover. The physician becomes a broker with the payer on behalf of his or her patient to obtain the needed services. Sometimes the patient becomes a broker between the physician and the payer when the two parties cannot resolve who is responsible for unpaid bills. And when a patient is unhappy with services, both the physician and payer can be targeted by the patient for legal intervention. The virtues of trust and loyalty valued in the dyadic relationship of the past have been replaced by what is expedient and self-serving in a triad in which all parties must prove themselves to each other.

More health care decisions are being made bureaucratically. Bureaucratization shifts decisions away from the patient toward the physician, away from the physician to the organization, and away from the organization to a conglomerate. More and more diagnoses and prognoses are formulated by a series of people and teams in a process in which the power to act is funneled through a bureaucratic structure. No one person is in control and follow-up often falls through the cracks. Therefore it is not surprising that some health providers have left their profession for other employment. Other providers remain and try to subvert the existing system of care.

A survey of internists in eight cities found that 45 percent of the physicians considered it ethical to deceive insurance companies and HMOs in order to secure payment for treatment when patients cannot obtain it another way (Freeman et al. 1999). Most of the physicians (76 percent) believed that their primary professional responsibility is to practice as their patient's advocate. The more potentially lifesaving the coverage, the stronger the support for lying. The physician as a broker of health care is often conflicted when he or she has to compromise what the physician knows would be a better treatment for a patient with the treatment that a payer will approve and pay for.

Health Care: Managing a "Tough" Culture

Health care has become an increasingly tough culture (Bruhn 2001b). Cultures are judged as tough or easy depending on the ways and means (paths) they provide for their members to meet their needs. The core of a culture is its set of values. The value driving managed care is cost control; the value that health care professionals emphasize is providing quality care to the sick. Tough cultures are concerned with treating everyone the same whereas easy cultures focus on meeting the needs of individuals. The values held by the managers of care conflict with those held by the providers of care. Since values cannot be managed, the boundaries protecting these two sets of opposing values frequently produce a great deal of tension and conflict. The patient is often forgotten in the process of negotiating win/lose outcomes. There is no evidence that either managers or providers will change their values or become more flexible in negotiating their respective boundaries. Therefore managers and providers need to become more skilled in managing conflict.

This book helps the reader understand the social and psychological aspects of territoriality and turfism and gives a range of examples and vignettes to illustrate the dynamics of boundaries among health professionals, and between health professionals and others with whom they interact both inside and outside the health care conglomerate. Because the organization and delivery of health care is constantly being bombarded by social change, boundaries are continually being modified. It takes work to keep boundaries flexible or rigid and is therefore impossible to provide the reader with a boilerplate of actions to manage boundaries in all types of organizations or situations. Guidelines and procedures for arbitration and mediation are useful in helping to resolve many conflicts, the most difficult of which focus on values. Values cannot be debated since individuals develop values based on their own history and interests.

Managers and providers must work to seek ways so that all legitimate values in an enterprise can be served. Health professionals value autonomy but autonomy is impossible under managed care. On the other hand, managed care decision makers often seem to make autonomous judgments about the importance or relevance of various health care procedures about which they have no training. It would seem that costs can be contained and quality care delivered if both parties agree that the patient should be the focus. A health care system that is less adversarial would benefit providers, payers, and patients alike, and perhaps all parties would feel more satisfied with their outcomes.

References

Bruhn, John G. 2001a. "Equal Partners: Doctors and Patients Explore the Limits of Autonomy." *Journal of the Oklahoma State Medical Association* 94:46–54.

Bruhn, John G. 2001b. "Managing Tough and Easy Organizational Cultures." *Health Care Manager* 20:1–10.

Freeman, Victor G., Saif S. Rathorne, Kevin P. Weinfurt, Kevin A. Schulman, and Daniel P. Sulmasy. 1999. "Lying for Patients: Physician Deception of Third-Party Payers." *Archives of Internal Medicine* 159:2263–70.

Lewis, Bonnie L. and Dale F. Parent. 2001. "Health Care Equity." Pp. 293–311 in *Handbook of Clinical Sociology*, 2nd ed., edited by H. M. Rebach and J. G. Bruhn. New York: Kluwer Academic/Plenum Publishers.

John G. Bruhn
Harold Grumet Levine
Paula L. Levine

PREFACE

This book grew out of our observations and experiences while working in health science centers. The written literature contains relatively little about boundaries, territoriality, and turfism, yet these phenomena are at the root of many of the problems health professionals encounter.

All living beings establish territories, or spaces, which they dominate. These territories, which increase their chances of survival, have psychological as well as physical importance. Physical workspace is important in all occupations. The concept of space, and the defense of such space, are important phenomena in *all* human experience, that of the farmer in Frost's *Mending Wall,* and that of the corporate executive who covets a corner office.

Competition for space, both real and metaphysical, is rampant in the health professions. The rapid growth of knowledge and skill in preventing disease, and in diagnosing and managing illness, have led to an explosion of new health professions and an expansion and enrichment of old, established ones. Optimal exploitation of this expanded knowledge demands the cooperation and coordination of health professionals as well as a clear delineation of their functions. Unfortunately, conflicts, misunderstandings, and fear of competition often make it difficult to take advantage of the opportunities afforded by new knowledge and new technologies.

Turf and territoriality manifest themselves in the relationships among health professionals—how they work with each other, if at all, and how their interrelationships affect others, especially patients. Protecting one's professional turf is critical in the fields of health professions education and health care where innovations constantly create the need to learn new skills and new technologies. New types of professionals, who emerge in response to new technologies, in turn, wish to establish their identities and stake out their territories.

It is common for students in the various health professions to learn about working in teams to benefit the patient, but it is rare for those students to learn together or to learn about what others do. Specialization and protectionism are modelled by members of the faculty. Occasionally, however, an exceptional team does arise and function because of a unique mix of personalities with a common mission.

Administrators spend most of their time "getting people to work together, and keeping others apart." Boundaries will always exist; it is not our intention to suggest that they be eliminated. We propose to illustrate various types of boundary situations, issues, and guidelines for alleviating conflicts so that all may benefit from a more productive and satisfying workplace.

This text can be used by both students and professionals. Most health professions students lack experience in dealing with boundaries, and retain idealistic views of curing, healing, and solving. When they enter clinical situations, however, and experience the various environments provided by their internships, they experience the types of concepts, situations, and dilemmas described within this book.

The contents of this book can easily be applied to non-health work settings. Although we have focused on health care settings, we hope that administrators in other fields will derive insights and guidelines from this book that they can generalize to help them become effective and creative boundary managers.

Boundaries matter. Wherever they exist, they affect the behavior of decision makers and make it easier, or more difficult, to achieve collective goals. Hopefully, we can work together to bring about a world that contains fewer walls and more flexible fencelines.

JOHN G. BRUHN
HAROLD G. LEVINE
PAULA L. LEVINE

ACKNOWLEDGMENTS

We are grateful to Elena Cook who typed numerous drafts of the book. Geronimo Garcia helped design all of the figures and illustrations. Paula Levine provided expertise in editing, proofreading and preparing the index.

Aspen Publishers, Inc. gave us permission to reproduce parts of the following publications:

Bruhn, John G.: Managerial indecisiveness: When the monkeys run the zoo. *Health Care Supervisor*, 8(4): 55–64, 1990.

Bruhn, John G. Control, narcissism, and management style. *Health Care Supervisor*, 9(4): 43–52, 1991.

Bruhn, John G., and Lewis, Raymond: Boundary fighting: Territorial conflicts in health organizations. *Health Care Supervisor*, 10(4): 56–65, 1992.

CONTENTS

MANAGING BOUNDARIES
IN THE
HEALTH PROFESSIONS

Chapter 1

ABOUT BOUNDARIES

A line has been drawn in the sand.... Withdraw from
Kuwait unconditionally and immediately, or face the ter-
rible consequences.

George Bush
August 1990

Introduction

Boundaries keep people apart. Boundaries can be physical or psychological. Physical boundaries occupy space and limit access to separate spaces. Psychological boundaries tell us what we should or should
not do. An example of a physical boundary is the skin, which separates
the body from the outside world and enables the organs to function.
Psychological boundaries are not inert like physical boundaries. Psychological boundaries influence the attitudes and feelings of those who erect
the boundaries and those who are confronted by the boundaries. For
example, the boundaries of Black segregation deeply affected those who
imposed segregation and those who were segregated (Ellison, 1952;
Baldwin, 1962). They rendered Blacks "invisible" to Whites and afflicted
Blacks with deep-seated feelings of inadequacy and anger, which have
gravely injured the ability of many Black people to grow and develop
fully as individuals.

Modern society is built upon a division of labor. Division of labor
erects work barriers, both behavioral and psychological, between all our
activities. These work barriers are essential for maintaining our complex
economic system. On the other hand, division of labor, the great source
of late 20th century productivity and wealth, requires teamwork and
cooperation among diverse groups of workers. Teamwork and cooperation are essential to the functioning of health care technology. However,
boundaries that facilitate a division of labor can also inhibit cooperation.

Boundaries exist among, between, and within nations, social institutions,

3

organizations, groups and individuals. This book will focus primarily on the social and psychological boundaries that exist in health institutions, such as hospitals, health science centers, and schools that educate health professionals. We are particularly interested in the ways in which boundary behavior impacts on the effectiveness of these institutions in carrying out their goals, on their responsiveness to meeting societal needs, and on their adaptability to social change. Our purpose is to examine and analyze boundary behavior in health institutions, to suggest practical ways in which boundaries can be better managed to facilitate an institution's productivity and contributions to society, and to suggest ways in which individual employees of health institutions can better realize their potential for professional growth in optimally managed workplaces. It is our premise that the inability to utilize the positive effects and minimize the negative effects of boundaries interferes with individuals, institutions, and indeed, nations, in their efforts to meet their goals and aspirations.

Several points should be emphasized at the outset. Boundaries are a part of being human and will always exist. We do not assume that all boundaries can be positive and facilitative, or damaging and inhibiting, nor do we presume to have an answer or a blueprint for managing or solving all boundary problems. Boundary issues must be recognized and managed by those who know the unique situations in which they occur, their history, and the players. We hope to provide the reader with a better understanding of boundary behavior, the purposes that boundaries serve, and the effects of boundaries on people.

Sources of Boundaries

The sources of boundaries and boundary problems lie within the nature of human beings, the methods we use to generate wealth, and the history and traditions we bring to the tasks of daily living. As McCrone (1991) points out, humankind is unique in that each of us has a strong sense of individuality, nurtured by our self-awareness, developed over many millenia by the spoken and, more recently, written language. As primates, we are intensely social animals. Our self-awareness makes us desire to "fit in" among our peers, but still stand out as individual and important. Our evolutionary heritage also makes us intensely territorial.

Territoriality

Aristotle and Pliny noted the demarcation and defense of territories by male birds, and the phenomenon was rediscovered sporadically through the first centuries of modern science (Wilson, 1975). The concept of territory has two referents—the restriction of behavior to a limited area, and defense of the area. The classic territory is an area, the boundaries of which are rigidly defended against cospecific individuals. In the broad sense, territoriality can be the actual defense of an area, which includes patrolling its boundaries and actively seeking out intruders; adherence to a home range coupled with aggression toward outsiders; and adherence to a home range with mutual avoidance between groups (Hinde, 1974).

The modern study of territory began in 1868 when Bernard Altum suggested that animals do not act, they are acted upon; they respond to drives and stimuli, including the territorial drive. A lack of translation made Altum's work inaccessible to the English-speaking scientific community; therefore, similar ideas were derived independently by British ornithologists. The term "territory" was introduced in 1903 by C. B. Moffat.

Territoriality is present in a number of species. In order to be so widespread and persistent, it must convey an evolutionary advantage. Probably, the development of territoriality diminished acts of aggression among animals and facilitated survival and reproduction. Examples of territorial behavior in humans abound in a variety of settings (Van Den Berghe, 1977).

The question of whether territorial tendencies are inborn or learned is unresolved. However, the widespread existence of territorial behavior in animals, including humans, seems to indicate that the drive for territory and personal space is characteristic of a number of species and of human societies. However, the variety of ways in which the drive for territory manifests itself indicates that behavior problems related to territoriality are based, to a great degree, on individual experiences and can be modified through learning. It is possible to teach cats, dogs, birds, and rats to live together in peace if the conditions in which they are raised are properly manipulated (Kuo, 1960).

In human societies, individuals and groups strive to establish and maintain territories to which access is limited, and the conventions of personal space are observed during social interaction. The clearest expression of the role of territoriality, as well as several interesting observations regarding territoriality, emerge from the literature on hunter-gatherer societies (Gold, 1982). Territoriality was most likely to predominate when resources were abundant. Sharing in bad times was not purely altruistic. Rivalries were channeled into things other than land. Tribes or groups defended the boundaries of the group rather than those of the territory. The most important facet of territoriality was its creation of a stable framework for the orderly conduct of everyday life. Some groups aggressively maintained sharply defined boundaries, but others were content with loosely defined territories and weakly defended peripheries. Thus, the potential range of boundary and territorial response was considerable.

The complexity of behavioral response to territorial issues was compounded when man became an urban animal. The dwelling supplied a physical and social territory. The neighborhood offered a type of social organization and exclusiveness based on a variety of elements, including socioeconomic factors, language, and culture. Cities provided different layouts and designs to give residents a sense of community. The social climate of cities provided anonymity. However, humans, who are confined within areas with growing populations and increasing densities, are forced to endure the shrinking of their personal physical space. When others become intolerably close, and there are no means of escape, aggressive behavior becomes increasingly probable. Veness (1964) suggests that close crowding by others may arouse concern for one's identity.

The expression of territoriality is a social construct. It can take different forms in different geographical and historical circumstances, and its manifestations must be understood within a specific context. The protection of personal space can fill some psychological needs, which, however, can be satisfied in a variety of contexts. In designing educational, service, and social institutions, we must recognize the intense need of humans to maintain control of their environment at the same time we recognize that a variety of organizational patterns, which meet human needs, can exist, but only some of these patterns are facilitative of the organizational mission.

Territory is the area of life that humans experience as their own, the area in which they exercise control, take initiatives, display expertise, or accept responsibility. It is the realm in which people enjoy a sense of independence and feel free to act on their own initiative (Brown, 1987; Bakker and Bakker-Rabdau, 1973). There are three broad types of human territory: tribal (public), family (home), and personal (body). Each nation flies its own flag, a symbolic embodiment of its territorial status. People, however, are not fully satisfied by membership in a large conglomeration of individuals, despite a shared territorial defense, so they form smaller, more personal subgroups—the club, the gang, the union, the fraternity or sorority, the social clique, the professional organization. Typical of all of these groups is the use of territorial signals—badges, banners, slogans, and other signs of group identity. Each of these modern tribes sets up its unique home base. In extreme cases, non-members are excluded, in others they are accepted as visitors with limited rights under a control system with special rules. At the heart of the specialized territories is a powerful feeling of security and importance, a sense of shared defense against the outside world.

The family (home) territory is the one in which humans feel most secure. When people enter a family's space, they sense that they must ask permission to do the simple things that they would consider a right elsewhere. Family territory is marked by numerous objects that indicate a family's uniqueness and history. A family unit, venturing out into the world, loads the car with its personal belongings and its territory becomes temporary and portable. The same territorial behavior is evident wherever family groups are clustered, e.g., parks, beaches.

Territorial behavior that is natural for the home often is inappropriate in the workplace. Work has a different purpose than family life. It profits extensively from the blending of a variety of talents. Talented people who are brought together at the worksite have different histories, interests, and cultures, while families and social groups are bound together by their similarities. Families and social groups enforce unexpressed codes of behavior because predictability and shared values are important in social interactions. People in the workplace may not share values and may not act in predictable ways.

Personal or body boundaries are those encompassed by the anatomical space of the body. Each person exercises rights over both his internal and his external bodily space. Goffman (1971) discusses eight territories of the self. He notes that the higher the social rank, the greater the size of all territories of the self and the greater the control across boundaries. Cultural factors, however, make status differences in the use of personal or body space more complex (Lyman and Scott, 1967–68).

Personal boundaries are essential for psychological stability. However, in instances of psychopathology, boundaries that have become extreme, either too porous or too rigid, may lead to defensiveness and loneliness (Paris, 1985). Extreme personal boundary behavior will usually result in the labeling of a person or group as "deviant," indicating that the behavior has crossed the boundary of what is considered acceptable (Lauderdale, 1976).

Personal opinions about morality and ethics and about what constitutes moral and ethical behavior, oft-times directly expressed on bumper stickers of cars and on T-shirts, are indicators of people's personal boundaries. In our society, we categorize and label people on the basis of their opinions as well as on their behavior. Labeling helps us to maintain some semblance of order and control in our personal lives vis-a-vis the larger society. However, it can also make it difficult for those who are labeled to work with those who are doing the labeling. Inappropriate labeling and stereotyping sometimes make it difficult for professionals, e.g., physicians and nurses, to work together. Such difficulties are compounded by gender differences and class differences.

Moral boundaries are difficult to monitor because it is not always obvious when they are being threatened unless, of course, an overt attempt is made to change a boundary. Moral and physical boundaries together form the totality of body or personal boundaries—the psychological, spiritual, and anatomical space of the body.

Lyman and Scott (1967–68) discuss another type of territory, the interactional territory, in which social gatherings, such as parties, occur. Every interactional territory makes a claim of boundary maintenance for the duration of the interaction. Interactional territories characteristically are mobile and fragile. The fragility of interactions is constantly being tested by newcomers and parvenus. Knowles (1972) found that dyads of different sex compositions respond differently to interactional boundaries, suggesting that the strength of the interactional boundary is not uniform; it varies with the characteristics of the interaction or unit. Male-female dyads were most protective of their social space, female-female dyads were next most protective, and male-male dyads were least protective. Sommer and Becker (1971) argue that an ecological perspective requires "concepts of people-in-situations" rather than of people on one hand and situations on the other. Space usage is affected by the social relationships among the users. In human affairs, territorial boundaries are continually under stress; borders can move inward or outward.

Personal Space

An individual not only claims physical space as his own, he has definite perceptions and feelings about his personal space, the invisible barrier that surrounds each of us and is demonstrated by the space we keep between ourselves and others (Hall, 1966). Sommer (1969) says that the best way to learn the location of invisible boundaries is to keep walking until somebody complains. We experience violations of our personal space almost daily, by the person in the cafeteria who pushes our tray along the serving line, the person in the grocery store who shoves us in the back with a grocery cart, the hurried driver who cuts sharply in front of us, causing us to brake suddenly, the person who comes early, one morning, to the gym and occupies our favorite treadmill, or the person who stares at us in a shopping mall—in all of these situations, we feel agitated because our personal space has been violated. Personal space is not necessarily spherical in shape, nor does it extend equally in all directions. People are better able to tolerate the close presence of a stranger beside them than in front of them (Sommer, 1969). We construct an "internal boundary" regarding what we consider to be "our" territory. We send signals to alert others to the limits of our territory. Most of the time, these signals are recognized and heeded, but, sometimes, an invader of our space precipitates a conflict. When people from cultures with divergent views of personal space try to communicate, trouble often begins. If an individual loses part of his territory, or sees an unsurmountable obstacle that limits his expansion, he may respond with aggression.

Bakker and Bakker-Rabdau (1973), take the position that an individual handles his territorial inclinations in accordance with three principles. Depending on his learning, his resources, and his interpretation of a situation, an individual may choose many different courses of action, ranging from unleashing an acid tongue to using brute force, in dealing with territorial problems. Social learning to acquire the skills needed to hold one's own in society is a key influence in the development of territorial behavior.

Whether or not someone perceives that his/her territory is being invaded depends upon that person's perception of a total situation based upon his/her previous experiences. Territorial infringement is not always obvious, nor is it interpreted in the same way by all observers. The division of labor that accompanies most health practice in the

Figure 1-1. Types of Boundaries.

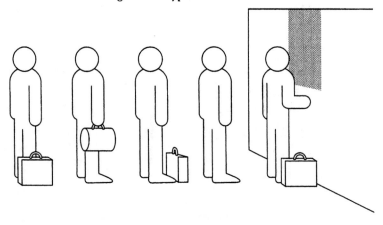

PHYSICAL BOUNDARIES

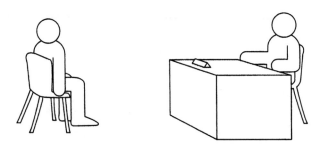

PSYCHOLOGICAL BOUNDARIES

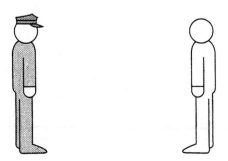

Source: John G. Bruhn   **SOCIAL BOUNDARIES**

professions, today, produces the metaphoric equivalent of a territory. The "expert" in an organization or community may believe that all problems relating to his specialty should be in his domain or territory. Thus, a pediatrician who moves to a community where most physicians are family physicians might expect the family physicians in the community to consult him about complex pediatric problems. However, the family physicians, who also are trained to treat children, might not feel the need to consult the pediatrician. Often, economic and historic issues intrude. Physical therapists who, historically, were trained by physician specialists (physiatrists), treat patients based upon a physician's prescription. Most family physicians and internists who send their patients to physical therapists know little about physical therapy and provide the therapists with little guidance, yet, in many states, physical therapists cannot treat patients without a physician referral, creating considerable territorial confusion and conflict.

Another principle involving one's territorial perceptions and behavior involves the availability to an individual of certain resources. For example, it is likely that a person who is alone and is approached by two strangers for directions will feel more apprehensive about the possible violation of his personal space than would a person who is with two other people. Having resources readily available to us usually makes us more tolerant of situations that might involve invasions of our space than we would be had we no resources to call upon. Regardless of its source, man has the capability to determine the way in which to handle his territorial impulse. (see Figure 1-1).

Territory can be distinguished from individual distance (social distance or personal space). Individual distance is the minimum distance that an animal routinely keeps between itself and other members of the same species. Paul Leyhausen used the following German fable to clarify the significance of individual distance.

> One very cold night a group of porcupines were huddled together for warmth. However, their spines made proximity uncomfortable, so they moved apart again and got cold. After shuffling repeatedly in and out, they eventually found a distance at which they could be comfortably warm without getting pricked. This distance they henceforth called decency and good manners (Wilson, 1975, p. 257).

Hall (1966) grasped the implication of this zoological principle for human beings and suggested the need for a discipline of "proxemics," the systematic study of the use of space as a specialized component of culture. Civilized man, Hall argued, uses walls to provide a sense of adequate space in his "unnaturally" dense habitations. Cultures differ markedly in their individual distances. Mediterranean peoples, including the French, tolerate closer packing in restaurants and other meeting places and stand closer to each other when speaking than do northern Europeans. An Englishman is likely to consider an Italian crude and forward, while the Italian may view the Englishman as cool and impolite.

Culture affects the ways in which we perceive and deal with our environment, that is, how we define turf and territory. In cultures where crowding is inevitable because of the shortage of space, cultural norms encourage defensiveness in regard to personal space. In short-term situations, we may permit greater tolerance of invasions of personal space than we do in those in which the situation is more prolonged, e.g., a crowded cable car in San Francisco or a crowded subway train in New York City will be tolerated according to the length of the ride. Crowding behavior in the United States usually is perceived as a violation of personal space, and is avoided if possible, whereas crowding and closeness in China is a way of life.

Hall (1959) notes that time, although it is a boundary, has different meanings and is handled differently in different cultures. In the United States, we earn it, save it, and waste it; in other cultures, time is experienced. Hall also discusses the language of space. Personal space, unlike territory, cannot be recognized by a marker. One's personal space is a function of factors, which include status, sex, age, and situation. Behavior relating to personal space is guided by an interaction between two or more individuals (Becker and Mayo, 1971). Where people stand in relation to each other signals their relationship and how they feel about each other. Keeping someone at "arm's length" is one way of expressing personal distance. The boundary line between an "arm's length" and touching varies in different cultures. Hall emphasizes that virtually everything we do is associated with the experience of space. Our sense of space is a synthesis of many types of sensory inputs that are molded and patterned by culture.

One of the most important questions that is deserving of future attention concerns the *basis* for the cultural and subcultural differences in personal space, spatial behavior, and reactions to crowding. Montagu (1971) provides a series of descriptions of early socialization practices relating to tactile behavior between parents and children of various cultural, subcultural, and socioeconomic groups. He advances the argument that every society has evolved unique ways of dealing with the child from the moment of its birth. It is on the basis of repeated sensory experiences of culturally prescribed stimulations that the child learns how to behave according to the requirements of its culture. He contrasts the impersonal childrearing practices of the English, Germans, and Americans with those of the more tactilely involved Latins, Russians, Jews, Japanese, implying the greater eventual preference that children of the former cultures will have, due to these practices, for larger spatial and psychological distances from other people than will children of the latter cultures. Aiello and Thompson (1980) believe that it is a combination of these early experiences *and* continued reinforcement of these experiences through interaction with the social and physical environment within one's culture that influences cultural differences in spatial preference. Since each of us superimposes a unique family culture upon the cultural milieu of our nationality, our individual boundary perceptions differ, creating a potential source of problems in education and at work.

Territoriality, whatever its source or its restrictions or blessings, allows a person to measure his personal assets against the norms of his reference group. His identity, security, and freedom are intimately tied to his territorial holdings—to paraphrase an old saying, territory makes the man (Bakker and Bakker-Rabdau, 1973).

Perceptions of Reality

Wilber (1981) points out that boundaries are illusions, products not of reality, but of the way we map and edit reality. People are always trying to bound their lives, their experiences, their realities. Therefore, every boundary line is a potential battle line. Boundaries are the invisible lines we draw to protect our personal identities and our personal resources. Testing the boundaries of others to determine who they are and how we should behave toward them is one of our most time-consuming activities.

Zerubavel (1992) says that we create islands of meaning. We place the objects we perceive in categories, separating them from each other. The perception of supposedly insular chunks of space is probably the most fundamental manifestation of our division of reality into islands of meaning. The way in which we divide time is evocative of the way we partition space. The manner in which we isolate space and time is manifested in the way we experience ourselves. Separateness is crucial to the development of selfhood. Boundaries make us feel secure.

There is no reason why entities should have only one fixed meaning. We do not have to choose between rigidity and fluidity. As Zerubavel notes, "We must therefore stop reifying the lines we draw and remember that the entities they help us define are only figments of our own mind" (p. 122).

An experiment described by Rosenhan (1973) provides a dramatic illustration of how we map and edit reality. Eight sane people secretly gained admission to 12 different mental hospitals. The pseudopatients and the nature of the experiment were not known to the hospital staffs. After calling the hospital for an appointment, each pseudopatient arrived at the admissions office complaining of hearing voices. No alterations of person, history, or circumstances, beyond the alleged symptoms and a false name, vocation, and employment were made. The pseudopatients were never detected as sane, and all, except one, were admitted to the hospitals with a diagnosis of schizophrenia. Failure to detect the deception during the course of hospitalization, which ranged from 7 to 52 days, may have been due to the fact that physicians operate with a bias, which statisticians call a type 2 error—they are more inclined to call a healthy person sick than a sick person healthy. It also indicates how we tend to operate based upon hidden assumptions. The physicians at the hospital were not prepared to deal with patients who lied about hearing voices. Their perceptions of reality did not include this possibility.

It was important to see whether the tendency to diagnose the sane as insane could be reversed. Another experiment was arranged at a research and teaching hospital where the staff had heard of the findings, but doubted that such an error could occur at their hospital. The staff were informed that at some time during the following three months, one or more pseudopatients would attempt to gain admission to the psychiatric hospital. Each staff member was asked to rate each patient who presented, at admission or on the ward, according to the likelihood that the patient was a pseudopatient. Judgments were obtained on 193 people who were admitted as psychiatric patients. Forty-one patients were alleged to be pseudopatients by at least one staff member, 23 were considered suspect by at least one psychiatrist, 19 were suspected by one psychiatrist and one other staff member. In actuality, no pseudopatients presented themselves during this period. Again, the staff had no experience with pseudopatients and no procedures for identifying such patients. The boundaries of their perceptions of reality did not include such patients until they heard about the experiment, and they did not have opportunities to test techniques for detecting such patients.

The experiment is instructive. It indicates that the definition of insanity is partly the result of a community's perception of reality. Phenomena such as insanity are partly based upon community consensus because insanity is usually inferred from behavior and often cannot be diagnosed by reference to physical changes in the brain. Health specialists once classified masturbation as a disease (Engelhardt, 1974) and only recently decided that homosexuality was not a mental illness (Bayer, 1987).

Also instructive is an illustration from history. Prior to World War II, it was considered acceptable to express racial and religious intolerance. Prestigious individuals argued, in respectable settings, that Jews should have limited access to education (Marden, 1952). No one imagined that a "civilized" nation would round up and murder millions of unarmed civilians, including women and children, simply because of their ethnic identity. Such "public" demonstrations of hatred have, as a result, lost respectability. Our definitions of what is acceptable and what is unacceptable keep changing as we uncover new facets of reality. The boundaries of our existence, in this age of rapid change, keep changing.

Milgram (1970) observed that when the inputs from our environment are too complex to process, we suffer from overload. We cannot establish priorities and choices. Life becomes a continuous set of encounters with overload. As Milgram points out, during the Genovese murder in Queens, New York, in 1964, 38 residents admitted to having witnessed part of the attack, but none went to the victim's aid or called the police. In a study devised to compare the willingness of city and town dwellers to assist strangers, Milgram found that city dwellers were less helpful due, in part, to the dangers inherent in living in a large city, such as Manhattan. It is significant that 75 percent of all city respondents received and answered messages by shouting through closed doors and peering out through peepholes; by contrast, 75 percent of the town respondents opened their doors.

As Milgram points out, all of us have cognitive maps of our environment; how we cope depends a great deal on what we perceive to be our options. These options are determined, in large part, by the boundaries we perceive in governing our behavior. When boundaries become blurred, adaptation becomes difficult because choices or options are unclear.

Development of Boundaries

As we have discussed, the development of psychological boundaries and territories is influenced greatly by the individual's social system and traditions. Some of the traditions inherited from past generations have lost their functions, but still have power to define boundaries and, therefore, territories.

Gender

Perhaps the most pervasive boundaries are those imposed by gender. In existing hunter-gatherer societies, women are burdened with pregnancy and the demands of infants (McCrone, 1991). They need male protection and food sharing. The males need females to provide sexual gratification and carry out domestic chores. These societies represent the probable division of labor in most primitive societies. Virtually all ancient societies were characterized by this type of gender boundary, although the nature of their boundaries varied. In most societies, males gained a virtual monopoly on positions of social power and influence, a condition that continued to exist until very recently, when the economic conditions that led to male dominance all but disappeared.

Male dominance has had striking effects on the health professions. Male obstetricians, during the 19th century, began to take control of labor and delivery from the female midwives, often to the detriment of women's health care (Leavitt, 1989; Eaton and Webb, 1979). Nursing and most of the allied health professions, with the notable exception of physician's assistants, have become dominated by females, a development that has contributed to the shortage of nurses as talented women pursue other professions (U.S. Bureau of the Census, 1991). These issues will be discussed in greater detail in later sections of this book.

Ethnic Differences

Another type of barrier is that due to ethnicity. Ethnic differences contribute to the cultural differences that lead to social norms. Since norms define boundaries, ethnic differences can lead to serious boundary problems.

Ethnic differences are often compounded by religious differences, language differences, and differences in history, physical appearance, social customs, and values. During the 19th and 20th centuries, powerful emotional appeals to nationalism were added to the witches' brew of ethnic differences. In some cases, discrimination based on ethnic differences produced economic gains. English landowners compiled great economic gains through the systematic repression, for almost 300 years, of Irish Catholics (Kee, 1982). White landowners in the Americas justified the repression of Black slaves on the premise that their ethnic differences made them "inferior" to Whites, yet the exploitation of these "inferior" people enabled the White landowners to earn a great deal of money.

The rise of capitalism has rendered boundaries due to ethnicity dangerous and unproductive. In a market society, inappropriate boundaries tend to stifle effectiveness and productivity. A talented ethnic group, the Jews, were feared and hated, for a variety of reasons that had little to do with their conduct, by many of the common people in Europe. However, the rulers and capitalists of many European nations, because they wished to encourage economic growth, acted to emancipate the Jews. The development of capitalism, thereby, facilitated the modern emancipation of the Jews (Rivkin, 1971).

Because of the social prestige of medicine, entrance into the medical profession was restricted to members of majority populations in most countries, while health occupations of low status, e.g., nurses' aides, licensed vocational nurses, became dominated by female members of ethnic minorities. Lack of representation in positions of power and prestige by minorities and women contributed to a lack of sensitivity to health care issues in minority populations. The infamous Tuskegee experiments on Blacks (Jones, 1981), who were left untreated for syphilis, and the failure of many clinical trials to include women (Healy, 1991), are examples of this problem.

Class and Hierarchy

Although hierarchies are necessary to the functioning of modern bureaucratic organizations, class systems and hierarchies can create inappropriate boundaries. The hunter-gatherer and pastoral societies of the past exhibited a strong desire for equality and fear of the inappropriate boundaries created by a class society. Many passages in the Hebrew Bible indicate the strong anti-hierarchical bias of the ancient Hebrews. A passage from the *First Book of Samuel* (8:16–20) suggests that it was only because the people of ancient Israel felt a strong need for protection from other nations that they created a monarchy led by warrior kings.

A thousand year old conflict, in which the conquerors gained landed estates and imposed a rigid class society, resulted in the evolution of modern England (Morgan, 1988). The secondary psychological advantages gained from membership in a privileged class greatly inhibited the ability of Britain's leadership to capitalize on the country's early gains in industrialization. The British military was handicapped by an excessive reliance on amateur leaders who had the right accent and connections, but were hopelessly inept. The system was satirized by Sir William Gilbert when he told of the office boy who "polished up the handle of the big front door . . . I polished up that handle oh so carefullee, That now I am the ruler of the Queen's Navee!" (1939).

The failures of British management led to the development of powerful unions, which regarded management as their enemy rather than as a partner in a common social enterprise (Johnson, 1991). This development was partially emulated in the United States where the disdain of management for the workers led to the creation of antagonistic unions. Rigid boundaries between various levels of a hierarchy, and the treatment of workers as production tools rather than as colleagues, led to lack of quality control, inefficient, and ineffective production. Ironically, the post-war Japanese went to American business schools to learn how to organize production and to avoid the inappropriate use of boundaries. Companies like IBM, under the leadership of the Watsons, father and son, have long been aware of the benefits of treating all employees with dignity and respect (Augarten, 1984).

Monopoly

Another source of boundaries is a result of economic advantage. The liberal economists of the 18th century, exemplified by Adam Smith, and their modern disciples, such as Milton Friedman, have taught us that allowing any group or organization to gain a monopoly, in which boundaries enclose economic activity, is deleterious to the effectiveness of the enterprise and the public interest (Berlant, 1975). Monopolistic or semi-monopolistic enterprises tend to resist new ideas and become preoccupied with bureaucratic goals rather than serve the public. Examples abound, such as the decline of the American steel industry when relying on tariffs rather than working to develop innovations to meet the challenges of international competition damaged its competitiveness (Glastris, 1989). Monopolies are sometimes necessary because of issues of feasibility, e.g., it's desirable to have only one local phone company, and private armies might interfere with the overall mission of our government's armed forces to protect our country.

Licensed professions are legal monopolies granted by the government to selected groups of individuals who have completed certain educational requirements and passed licensure examinations. Thus, professional licensure creates boundaries that are enforced by State penalties (Berlant, 1975). Sometimes, quasi-licenses are developed by practitioners of occupations that are not licensed through the establishment of certification programs based upon educational and experiential requirements. For example, laboratory technicians and technologists may not be licensed, but laboratories are required by certain regulatory groups to employ only certified employees, thereby giving the certificate the force and effectiveness of a license.

Licensure and certification provide important economic gains for those who possess the desired documents. A physician's power to prescribe drugs, which is enforced in the United States, but not in such countries as Mexico, has enormous economic implications. The patient must visit the physician at periodic intervals in order to obtain drugs and, thus, is forced to pay an advising fee as well as the price of the drug.

Other occupations and professions have coveted the legalized monopoly presented by physicians and have striven to come to terms with existing monopoly. For example, the pharmacists in England have ceded to the physicians the right to give advice about drugs and have tried, in return, to monopolize the right to dispense drugs (Berlant, 1975; Eaton and Webb, 1979). The monopolistic power of physicians has been justified on the grounds that it protects the public from quacks and charlatans and encourages members of the profession to seek the highest standards in education and practice (Berlant, 1975).

Since the goals of various professions are related to preserving the monopoly as well as to providing expert service to the public, it is often difficult for professionals in different specialties to work together. Professions resist internal divisions of labor that might disadvantage the majority of members of a profession. For example, the General Practitioners in the American Medical Association have resisted limitations on the practice of generalists. Theoretically, any graduate M.D. can practice surgery, although hospital policies and the threat of malpractice suits restrict most surgical practice, in the 1990s, to those who have gone through a surgical residency training (Starr, 1982, p. 357).

Professionally licensed or certified individuals resist bureaucratic divisions of labor because they can deprive them of jealously guarded privileges and control. In most job situations, management tries to develop work policies and guidelines that are based upon grounds of efficiency and effectiveness. These "rational" boundaries can be stymied by constraints created by licensure or certification procedures. For example, nursing has created a number of divisions, based on education, that can stymie good management. A graduate of a diploma nursing program may not be allowed to accept certain responsibilities delegated to a baccalaureate degree nurse, even though the specific nursing training of the two groups is similar; much of the extra time spent in educating the baccalaureate degree nurse is taken up by liberal arts courses (Riffle et al., 1985).

History and Tradition

Many boundary problems result from historical developments. For example, neurology and psychiatry have a common certifying board. The boundary issues relating to these distinct specialties were handled more effectively as the specialties developed than were those of other related groups of health professionals, for example, physiatry and orthopedic surgery, which have a different historical development. Psychiatric social workers, clinical psychologists, and psychiatrists often perform similar functions, but their training is different so that controversies emerge, e.g., the exclusive right of the psychiatrists to prescribe drugs.

It is natural for humans to develop psychological territories so that they can function effectively in performing the tasks of living, especially the tasks of performing one's occupational duties. In a perfectly rational world, the person's territory would be defined by his expertise and interests, and by the needs of society. However, gender, ethnicity, economic interests, including the desire for monopoly, and history influence one's personal definitions of territory and boundaries as well as the definitions imposed by the social and legal systems.

Purposes and Functions of Boundaries

Boundaries have a number of positive purposes: they guide us in situations where we feel uncertain about how we should behave; they permit us some leeway in personal creativity regarding how to behave in certain situations; they provide a degree of protection for our personal vulnerabilities; they reflect the strength of our personal values and beliefs, which help others to identify exceptional and different people for special tasks; they help us to control aggression in everyday life; they help us to respond more easily and rapidly to changes in our environment; and, in the workplace, they help us to define the level and breadth of our responsibilities. Boundaries also help us to take advantage of the assets we have developed, either through specialized training, experience, personal abilities, or through membership in powerful organizations by virtue of accidents of birth, e.g., gender, class, ethnicity.

Types of Boundaries

Hartmann (1991) points out that we create mental boundaries that are not absolute: they can be thick or solid or relatively thin or permeable. He believes that the thickness of boundaries is a dimension of personality. Hartmann states that some people are solid, well-organized and well-defended. Such people are "thick-skinned" and have thick boundaries. At the other extreme are people who are sensitive, open, or vulnerable. They experience different thoughts and feelings simultaneously. Such people have thin boundaries. Most people fit in between these extremes or have a mixture of boundaries.

The concept of mental boundaries is not new. William James discussed two types of temperament, rationalist and empiricist. Some of Freud's followers used the term, "ego boundary," and Carl Jung initiated considerable work on personality types. Hartmann has extended these earlier works in his approach to the measurement of mental boundaries as a new way to look at personality.

Developing Personal Boundaries

Animal studies indicate that individual distance is learned early. The human infant, at approximately six months of age, begins to attempt the process of separation-individuation from its mother; by age three, it has attained a fairly stable sense of self-boundaries (Mahler et al., 1975). At about age five, with the specific influences of school, family, peers, and the media, a child learns to broaden and solidify boundaries (Aiello, 1987). Developing personal boundaries involves an assessment of what others expect from one as well as one's own standards of behavior. The gap between self-other expectations establishes the outside limits of boundary perceptions. The continual testing of these self-other expectations in a variety of social situations helps young people to develop a system of values and their relative priorities. As individuals accumulate life experiences, they develop more stable sets of boundaries based on their values and beliefs.

Our boundary beliefs help to shape our values and the ways in which we view the world. This paradigm includes those behaviors that we have learned to be permissible and acceptable ways to solve life's problems. Different paradigms are advantageous because different persons may view the same information differently and make different suggestions. Sometimes, we become "fixed" in the views our individual paradigms provide and are unwilling to change. Similarly, our values, beliefs, and boundaries can become "fixed." Such rigid boundaries can limit our motivation to expand our horizons to accept new challenges and expectations. If we think that we cannot achieve certain goals because of lack of ability, we tend not to try (Atkinson, 1982). Sometimes, gender and ethnic identifications get in our way; we may believe that ethnic minorities do not do well in school or that girls cannot learn complicated mathematics.

Schaef and Fassel (1988) point out that just as there are individual addicts, organizations also can become addicted to their paradigms so that they are no longer responsive to the needs of the clients they propose to serve. Such organizations become addicted to power and control, become more isolated from society, and lose their sense of morality. When criticized, addictive organizations often become more rigid and defensive and fortify their boundaries, which, in turn, heightens their vulnerability to their critics. Professionals can adopt a view of their responsibilities that puts them into an adversarial role towards their clients. Teachers can have low expectations of their students' capabilities and inhibit the students' growth.

Some organizations are unable to adjust to the realities of a rapidly changing world. IBM had to be persuaded to embark on electronics by Thomas Watson, Jr. because the older managers were afraid that their customers would shy away from something so new and possibly unreliable. The executives at IBM later hesitated to get into computers because they were expensive. However, the defense initiatives established by the Korean War persuaded the company to move ahead and develop electronic computers. Later, in the 1970s, IBM was slow to respond to the rising interest in personal computers, initially failing, because of tunnel vision, to recognize the existence of a major new market (Augarten, 1984).

Perhaps the best example of fear of change occurred in the communist societies, which could not accommodate to the rapid social and economic changes of the post World War II world and fell helplessly behind to collapse in the late 80s and early 90s.

Financial pressures can lead to the adoption of policies that establish rigid boundaries regarding who can and cannot be served. Rather than attempt to mitigate the effects of these inappropriate boundaries, health professionals can become rigid and intolerant and see their roles as those of deciding on eligibility rather than those of helping their clients walk through the maze. Sometimes, the time pressures and resource limitations placed on health professionals cause them to develop inhumane attitudes toward patients, resulting in an almost complete reversal in the helpful attitudes desired in such professionals. *The House of God* (Shem, 1978) depicts the effects of such situations in physician training.

Boundaries and Social Norms

Norms are agreed upon standards or rules that govern our behavior. For example, it is a generally agreed upon norm that people do not go outside without their clothes on. There are designated areas, such as nude beaches, where nudity is permitted. Boundaries are personal interpretations of norms. For example, a person may wish to sunbathe nude in the privacy of his/her yard. A degree of freedom in violating norms exists as long as the values of others are not infringed upon. Indeed, some people may have very strict boundaries regarding nudity, even in the privacy of their homes. The most striking example of persons who seem to have few, if any, boundaries may be that of the hippies of the 1960s whose dress, language, and behavior deliberately violated social norms. Exploring the parameters of "no boundary awareness" through the aid of drugs was the ultimate insult to societal norms. Hippies were seeking to define their values and identities through the defiance of traditional norms. It is possible that an individual's boundary for a given behavior is more strict or liberal than society's norm. It is the degree to which individuals adhere to normative behavior that determines their social acceptability. Individuals tend to affiliate with other individuals and groups who share similar boundary perceptions.

The workplace offers many examples of the interplay between norms and boundaries. The norm for a standard workday, in many places, is 8 a.m. to 5 p.m. with time off for lunch and periodic breaks. Most employees adhere to this norm; they call in or notify their boss in advance when they expect to be late, and usually offer to make up the time. Since smoke-free workplaces are now more common, smokers often have to go outside a building to smoke. Smokers often can be seen congregated outside an office building a few minutes before 8 a.m. to have a cigarette before starting work. While this behavior respects the boundary of a smoke-free building, in our place of work, we have observed that smokers stretch this boundary in taking smoking breaks. They seem to take more breaks than they did before the building was designated smoke free. Smokers have to take extra time to reach the ground floor of the building, and most of the "heavy" smokers have resisted programs to help them to reduce or quit smoking and take more breaks to smoke. Boundary issues become a problem when the total secretarial staff of an office, comprised of two or three secretaries, take a smoke break simultaneously. Phones go unanswered, faculty cannot be located, and a host of communication problems arise for several fifteen-minute periods during a workday. Other employees become aware of the behavior and become frustrated or angry when they are caught in one of the fifteen minute communication voids.

If there are a sufficient number of smokers in a workplace, smoking breaks can become an issue for managerial arbitration. Smokers already believe that their rights have been compromised by the prevailing dictum of the non-smoking majority. Non-smokers, on the other hand, believe that smokers are taking advantage of the smoke-free building policy. As Hirschhorn (1988) points out, a boundary can create anxiety when it creates destabilizing dependencies so that people are unable to accomplish their tasks, when it highlights people who are trying to accomplish their tasks, and when the boundary stimulates fear of one's own aggression and the aggression of others. Smokers may be accused by non-smokers of irresponsibility. The environment of the workplace and relationships among workers may become strained. This situation may exist for some time as each side retreats from an overt boundary clash; eventually, however, the quality of work and the morale of the workplace will become affected and an aggressive display may eventually erupt over a matter that is not even related to smoking behavior.

Management can create a clash between norms and boundaries unintentionally. A new chair of a psychiatry department in a medical school had come from a federal institution where the key administrator could implement ideas and programs without consulting with the rank and file. In a university environment, however, to begin a new program and obligate faculty to it, without warning or discussion, violates a sacred norm. Without consulting his colleagues, the chair instituted an anxiety hotline, assigned faculty to supervise its operation, and abruptly left town. While individual faculty members perceived the effects of this action differently, most felt that their boundaries had been violated.

Psychological boundaries are guidelines, adopted consciously or unconsciously, which help individuals control their environment to make it more manageable. Management often adopts policies, due to the exigencies of the workplace, which can be counterproductive. For example, adopting widespread anti-smoking policies may seem a reasonable attempt to deal with a pressing social issue. However, such a policy may have undesirable side effects. Boundaries develop from perceptions that call upon management to be insightful, sensitive, and adaptable to them. There is no way that all employees can achieve optimum satisfaction in a workplace. Yet, if employees individually and collectively *perceive* that management is sensitive to their needs, they are less likely to be divisive and non-productive. It is when employees' perceptions are ignored or badly managed that a workplace is characterized by turnover, low morale, bickering, and non-productivity.

Testing Boundaries with Labels

Labeling is a potent, yet subtle means by which individuals cross boundaries, learn new roles, and accept new identities. Scott (1969), in *The Making of Blind Men,* states that if a person is labeled blind by certain administrative criteria, he is likely to become enmeshed in care-giving agencies that encourage him to accept a definition of himself as helpless and to learn to play the role of the blind man.

Rosenhan (1973) argues that what is viewed as normal in one culture may be seen as aberrant in another. He indicates that the perception of behavior as schizophrenic is relative to context; once the label of schizophrenia has been applied, the diagnosis acts on patient, family, and relatives as a self-fulfilling prophecy. Eventually, the patient accepts the diagnosis and behaves accordingly.

Rivers (1926) analyzed the concept of death among the Melanesians. Persons who are seriously ill and likely to die, or who are too old, from the Melanesian point of view, and ready to die, are labeled with the word, *mate,* which means "dead person." They then become subjects of a degradation ceremony in which they are deprived of their rights, are perceived "as if dead," and then are literally buried alive.

Labels are indicators of boundaries in that they define how we are to respond to those who are labeled. Many of us need to label people to help simplify our lives and make the tasks of living in a community more manageable. Often, we use labels without directly experiencing the person or group being labeled. When this occurs, labeling can limit our experiences by depriving us of the opportunity to interact with a variety of personalities and can be destructive to the object of the label. Indeed, labels carry a potent social pressure to act according to the stereotype implied by the label. Thus, adolescents may be given a license, by the label, to be irresponsible and difficult.

Labels can prophesy what will happen to a person. As Allport (1954) noted, "the important property of a noun is that it brings many grains of sand into a single pail, disregarding the fact that the same grains might fit just as appropriately into another pail. The very act of classifying forces us to overlook other features. Every label applied to a person refers to only one aspect of his/her nature." Some labels, such as "blind man," "head injured," "crippled," are exceedingly salient and powerful (Bruhn, 1991). Sontag (1978) has described the potency of metaphors with respect to tuberculosis and cancer and the ways in which fantasies surrounding these diseases have flourished because they are associated with a specific outcome.

Recently, one of us adjudicated a grievance by an occupational therapy student who perceived that he was being dismissed from a program, in large part, because he was being labeled. The student, who had suffered a closed head injury in a car accident, had been rehabilitated, but had some residual difficulty in processing and prioritizing information, especially when much information was presented rapidly. He needed some structure and found that frequent, immediate feedback from others helped him to sharpen his short-term memory. The Texas Rehabilitation Commission found him to be a worthy and capable candidate for entering a health occupation. After applying and being admitted, in a competitive process, to a baccalaureate allied health program, the student achieved a 3.1 average in his didactic courses. In his last year of study, when he was ready to go off campus on his clinical preceptorship, a faculty member said, "I hope you pass." The student did not perform satisfactorily in his three month clinical experience and was criticized by his clinical supervisors for "inappropriate behavior" and "not remembering verbal instructions," which put some patients at risk of injury. The faculty member who arranged a second, more extended clinical placement for the student told the clinical instructors that the student was a "slow learner," supposedly to justify the longer than usual placement. After a second unsatisfactory experience, the student's department recommended his dismissal from the program. When the student commented to a faculty member in the department that he did not believe the practitioners at the clinical site should have been told that he was a "slow learner," the faculty member replied, "But that's better than telling them you had a head injury!"

Intervention by the Dean of the school empowered the department to arrange two more clinical experiences, of standard length and with no pre-labels to be given to the practitioners at the sites, for the student. The student has since graduated following the satisfactory completion of these experiences.

Pre-labels color people's expectations. Instructors at clinical sites need some information about a student's medical history in order to prevent potential problems for the student and the clinical sponsor, but perhaps the student should be the one to tell his clinical supervisors what he wishes them to know about his personal and medical history. Certainly, each student with a disability is unique in respect to his/her experience with the disability. Astute clinicians should be able to discern the strengths and weaknesses of students without predetermined labels. Sponsors, however, must consider the welfare of their patients, and are sensitive to possible malpractice situations.

This case raises obvious legal and ethical dilemmas regarding the rights of students who have disabilities and indicates how information about their disabilities, which might be thought to be helpful, can actually be detrimental to their learning. In some cases, the label suggested by a diagnosis of a closed head injury, diabetes, or dyslexia may cause faculty and fellow students to limit their expectations concerning a student's performance. If the student performs badly because he or she is expected to perform badly, a great waste of human potential has occurred. Nevertheless, "slower than normal" responses, in the absence of information about a student's disability, might suggest poor motivation or ability. Perhaps, clinical supervisors should be given information about "exceptional" or "different" students so that they may provide such students with extra attention, supervision, or other modifications of their programs to facilitate their learning. Yet, information deemed to be helpful can also be harmful. As health professionals, we take pride in recognizing the individual needs of patients and in crafting their treatment and rehabilitation to meet those needs. The labels we so freely use to categorize people in our work can become so much a part of us that we become unaware of the subtle, yet devastating effects of these labels when they are used outside a treatment context. The use of diagnostic labels has its place, but the inappropriate and insensitive use of labels can be more disabling than a disability.

The health professions, supposedly, are receptive to entertaining applications from disabled and handicapped students, but it is not certain that health professions schools and faculties are really willing to take seriously the special needs of these students or to deal with the vexing issues in terms of labels and the need to safeguard patients treated by such students.

Health Boundaries

How people express or show their values, feelings, and beliefs regarding health and illness is a form of language that is culturally unique. Indeed, symptoms have to be decoded in order to be understood by the health professional. Not only what a patient says, but how he says it and what he does not say are important in understanding health and illness behavior.

Pliskin (1987) explores the cultural confrontation and misunderstandings that exist between Israeli health care professionals and the large number of Iranian immigrants who seek medical help. Her findings illuminate the problem of crosscultural communication as well as add to our knowledge of the culture of each group. Pliskin argues that medical institutions, language, and treatment are socially and culturally constructed. When patterns of meanings, beliefs, and social interactions differ between doctor and patient, problems of interpretation can occur. This is vividly illustrated in Israel, where clinicians have difficulty understanding the complaints of their Iranian patients and have coined a term to describe a supposedly culture-bound disorder associated with Iranians, "Parsitis," or the Persian syndrome. Pliskin explains the clinical problem of "Parsitis" by examining cultural differences, which create silent boundaries between therapists and patients and cause both to become frustrated by the clinical encounter (Murphy, 1976).

It has been said that "people who speak different languages live in different worlds, not the same world with different labels attached" (Edgerton and Karno, 1971). Anthropological linguists have suggested that men's minds are shaped by the language they speak. Kolers (1971) has suggested that bilinguals may have duplicate stores of meaning so that some information is readily accessible only through the language in which it is acquired. Clinically relevant processes may suffer in translation, so a patient's anxiety may be bound to the language being spoken. Marcos and his colleagues (1973) explored the differences in the verbal component of behavior in a series of Spanish-American schizophrenic patients whose psychiatric ratings reflected significantly greater psychopathology when they were interviewed in English. The major finding was that such patients do act differently in ways that the English-speaking clinician is likely to associate with increased psychopathology. Given the different levels of psychopathology found in the two languages, the researchers speculated about the "true" condition of the patients. Clinicians should be aware that speaking across language barriers arouses a complex group of socially learned perceptions that color the patient's and clinician's behavior.

Boundaries are Changeable

Boundaries are not fixed, except in our minds. Opportunities for individuals and societies are restricted mainly by our perceptions of boundaries. A sex change operation is a dramatic example of a change in boundaries; a man entering the nursing profession or a woman becoming a physician is now less dramatic. The Deanship of a medical school in the United States is a boundary that only two women have crossed (Association of American Medical Colleges, 1991). Our personal perceptions of boundaries are constantly being confronted with new information created by social and technological change. Leaving a convent to marry and become a university professor was extremely rare in the 1950s (Baldwin, 1950), but it is the focus of a book on role exit published in the 1980s (Ebaugh, 1988).

Ebaugh (1988) states that most of us in today's world are exes in one way or another. We have exited a marriage, a career, a religious group, a voluntary organization, an institution, or a stigmatized role, such as that of an alcoholic, a drug user, or even a smoker. Exes have always been around: ex-doctor, ex-athlete, ex-executive, ex-nun, ex-convict, and so forth. The one thing that all exes have in common is that they have crossed boundaries. Each has disengaged from a role that was central to his/her self-identity and reestablished an identity in a new role.

Even ethnic boundaries are not impermeable. Haaland (1969) describes how members of one tribe can change their ethnic identity to that of another by changing their method of making a living. The movie, *Europa, Europa* (Holland, 1990), based upon the autobiography of Solomon Perel, tells the story of a teenage Jewish boy who escaped Nazi arrest by assuming a false identity, even enrolling in the Hitler Youth corps.

Boundary changing is becoming commonplace in our society of second careers, women in the workforce, and single parent families. Equal opportunity and affirmative action have helped ethnic minorities, women, the handicapped, and the elderly to cross boundaries that previously were closed to them.

While social and technological change have helped to create opportunities and a need to open some boundaries, the major reason for boundary change is a change in our individual perceptions. In attempting to explain what causes our perceptions to change, Gene Amdahl, founder of Amdahl Corporation and Acys, Ltd., said, "I think it's impossible to really innovate unless you can deal with all aspects of a problem. If you can only deal with yolks or whites, it's pretty hard to make an omelette" (Kanter, 1983, p. 156). It is easier to hold on to our perceptions of boundaries when we have only limited information or refuse to consider other available information. Limited information is reinforcing to one's beliefs if that is all that is available. On the other hand, more information does not necessarily mean that individuals or countries will automatically discard old perceptions for new ones. There is a need to test expanded boundaries through experience. Experience helps to modify perceptions. It took American automobile manufacturers several years to realize that the way to compete against the sale of Japanese cars in the United States was not to limit their importation, but to improve the quality of American cars.

Kanter (1991, p. 151) states,

> For much of the twentieth century, business managers around the world confronted a series of walls. Walls between nations that establish the boundaries of national markets, national practices, or national social, economic, and political systems. Walls between the company and the society in which it exists, drawing sharp distinctions between corporate interests and social interests. Walls between work and home ... walls within the workplace itself ... and

walls between the company and its stockholders . . . Now we are told, the walls are crumbling.

In November 1990, *Harvard Business Review* conducted a world leadership survey in 25 countries to explore the boundaries of business. Boundaries within organizations were found to be shifting slowly, but the blurring of external boundaries is happening much faster. Customer service is the top success factor in nearly every country. Product quality is also ranked highly. The more joint venture experiences respondents had, the more they identified managerial issues as worrisome. For instance, Belgians were concerned about the loss of control in collaborative ventures. In contrast, Austrians, who report less joint venture activity, consider the biggest risks to be political factors and exchange rates. Corporate culture clashes are sure to be a prominent concern as the world creates a bigger agenda for business. "There are more cultures to understand, more time pressures to juggle, and more relationships to rethink" (Kanter, 1991). One inevitability of boundary change is the creation of new relationships, new roles, and new identities, all of which create new boundary agendas. Experience will tell which boundaries will be temporary and which will become more permanent.

In contrast to the rapidly changing boundaries of business, the social transformation of medicine and health care still are evolving, slowly and painfully (Starr, 1982). Two of the most pressing issues of medicine, which began emerging in the 1990s, are those of moral and economic problems. Rising costs have brought medical care under critical scrutiny, and the federal government has increasingly intervened in numerous ways. Scientific and technological progress have brought about a multitude of choices for each individual about how we live and how we die (Stein, 1978).

Medical care in America appears to be in the early stages of a major transformation to an institutional structure. The profession has long been able to resist corporate competition and corporate control by virtue of its collective organization, authority, and strategic position in mediating the relation of patients to hospitals, pharmaceutical companies, and use of third party payments. Today, physicians still hold authority and strategic positions, but these have eroded (Starr, 1982). The 1960s and 1970s broke down the uniformity and cohesiveness of the profession. In addition, the profession is no longer steadfastly opposed to the growth of corporate medicine. Physicians' commitment to solo practice has been eroding. Longer residency training cultivates group-oriented attitudes.

The rise of corporate medicine will restratify the profession. Professional autonomy will be lessened by the increasing corporate influence over the rules and standards of medical work. A corporate sector in health care is also likely to aggravate inequalities in access to health care. As Starr (1982, p. 448) notes, "This turn of events is the fruit of a history of accommodating professional and institutional interests, failing to exercise public control over public programs, then adopting piecemeal regulation to control the inflationary consequences, and, finally, cutting back programs and turning them back to the private sector."

The most salient aspect of medical organization is the enormous growth of specialization and subspecialization. While much of this development is due to the growth of biomedical science and technology, specialization is also a political process, bringing economic advantage and greater control over one's work and responsibilities (Stevens, 1971). Specialization, moreover, allows physicians to dominate a specified domain and to restrict competition (Mechanic, 1977). Because of the continuous development of new knowledge and the need for a defined universe, for purposes of continuing education, specialization is an essential element of modern medical practice. Specialization naturally sets boundaries around the types of problems to be considered by each health professional. However, specialization can bring with it a host of problems. The patient can be conceived by the health professional as a collection of signs and symptoms rather than a real person. Specialists are often unaware of the effects of treatments on organ systems that are not within their specialty. For example, medication prescribed by a cardiologist treating hypertension may cause impotence. As the number of specialties grows, the need for coordination can eventually destroy the gains in productivity accruing from the division of labor that led to specialization.

While specialization has affected many issues in medicine, the issue of greatest importance is the distinction between physicians who engage in primary, secondary, and tertiary levels of care. Each of these levels of care tends to be associated with particular modes of physician-patient interaction, settings of care, and extensiveness of care rendered. As health care administrators and government officials attempt to tighten expenditures by moving to a system of explicit rationing, intrusions into these boundaries of levels of care become commonplace. While physicians have retained considerable autonomy, the shift to the bureaucratization of medicine will modify the total framework of health services and how they are provided.

The bureaucratization of medicine also has the effect of diluting the personal responsibility of the provider. The interests of the patient, as well as others, will prevail. As this boundary of responsibility changes, it is likely that physicians will be more protective of their interests and rights. Many of the decisions relegated to physicians in the past, such as those regarding euthanasia and abortion, now involve laymen.

The power behind technological control over life and death increasingly is involving non-scientists. Several states have non-physicians on medical licensing boards, and review boards monitoring adverse reactions to prescription drugs include lawyers and consumer advocates. Public accountability is changing the boundaries of decision-making in medicine. Medical decisions are seldom strictly medical and involve some judgments for which physicians have no special training or authority (Stein, 1978). In addition, the lay public and medical practitioners are becoming increasingly aware of the limitations of the biomedical model of disease and its treatment. Wildavsky (1977, p. 105) has stated that, "According to the Great Equation, medical care equals health. But the Great Equation is wrong. More available medical care does not equal better health . . . whether you live, how well you live, and how long you live is 90 percent determined by factors over which doctors have little or no control." There has been a resurgence of interest in prevention and in the responsibility of individuals for their own state of health, bringing about greater demands by the public for health professionals who go beyond the boundary of illness care, for which they were trained, to offer guidance, advice, and information about how to keep one's health and how to increase the quality of one's life.

Modern health care's need for a team approach to the delivery of care is now achieving recognition (Nagi, 1975). This is especially true in the fields of rehabilitation and geriatrics where a number of professionals, such as physical therapists, occupational therapists, nurses, and social workers, as well as physicians must develop cooperative approaches to the management of patient care.

All of these initiatives, most of which have arisen outside the boundaries of medicine, have impacted on the education of health professionals, their practices, and the delivery of health care. The managers of health institutions and organizations are being called upon to seek new ways to manage boundaries and to instigate boundary changes. It will be increasingly more difficult for health educators and managers to separate professional responsibility from public accountability. We need to think about all of the conscious and unconscious boundaries that exist in the education of health care providers and in the provision of health care and to challenge the assumptions that underlie the system.

REFERENCES

Aiello, John R.: Human spatial behavior. In Stokols, Daniel and Altman, Irwin (eds.): *Handbook of Environmental Psychology.* Vol. 1. New York, Wiley, 1987.

Aiello, John R. and Thompson, Donna E.: Personal space, crowding, and spatial behavior in cultural context. In Altman, Irwin, Rapoport, Amos, and Wohlwill, Joachim F. (eds.): *Human Behavior and Environment: Advances in Theory and Research.* Vol. 4. New York, Plenum, 1980.

Allport, Gordon Willard: *The Nature of Prejudice.* Cambridge, Addison-Wesley, 1954.

Altum, Bernard: *Der Vogel und sein Leben.* Munster, W. Neimann, 1868.

Association of American Medical Colleges: Personal communication, 1991.

Atkinson, John W.: Motivational determinants of thematic apperception. In Stewart, Abigail J. (ed.): *Motivation and Society.* San Francisco, Jossey-Bass, 1982.

Augarten, Stan: *Bit by Bit: An Illustrated History of Computers.* New York, Ticknor & Fields, 1984.

Bakker, Cornelia B. and Bakker-Rabdau, Marianne K.: *No trespassing! Explorations in human territoriality.* San Francisco, Chandler & Sharp, 1973.

Baldwin, James: *Nobody Knows my Name: More Notes of a Native Son.* New York, Dell, 1962.

Baldwin, Monica: *I Leap Over the Wall.* New York, Signet, 1950.

Bayer, Ronald: *Homosexuality and American Psychiatry: The Politics of Diagnosis.* Second edition. Princeton, Princeton University Press, 1987.

Becker, Franklin D. and Mayo, Clara: Delineating personal distance and territoriality. *Environment and Behavior, 3:* 375–381, 1971.

Berlant, Jeffrey Lionel: *Profession and Monopoly: A Study of Medicine in the United States and Great Britain.* Berkeley, University of California Press, 1975.

Brown, Barbara B.: Territoriality. In Stokols, Daniel and Altman, Irwin, (eds.): *Handbook of Environmental Psychology.* Vol. 1. New York, Wiley, 1987.

Bruhn, John G.: Commentary: Nouns that cut: The negative effects of labelling by allied health professionals. *Journal of Allied Health, 20:* 229–231, 1991.

Eaton, Gail and Webb, Barbara: Boundary encroachment: Pharmacists in the clinical setting. *Sociology of Health and Illness, 1:* 69–89, 1979.

Ebaugh, Helen Rose Fuchs: *Becoming an Ex: The Process of Role Exit.* Chicago, University of Chicago Press, 1988.

Edgerton, Robert B. and Karno, Marvin: Mexican-American bilingualism and the perception of mental illness. *Archives of General Psychiatry, 24:* 268–290, 1971.

Ellison, Ralph: *The Invisible Man.* New York, Random House, 1952.

Engelhardt, H. Tristram, Jr.: The disease of masturbation: Values and the concept of disease. *Bulletin of the History of Medicine, 48:* 234–248, 1974.

First Samuel, 8:11–20. In: *The Holy Scriptures. According to the Masoretic Text.* Philadelphia, Jewish Publication Society, 1966.

Gilbert, Sir William S.: H.M.S. Pinafore. In: *Authentic Libretti of the Gilbert and Sullivan Operas.* New York, Crown, 1939.

Glastris, Paul: Steel's hollow comeback. *U.S. News and World Report, 106:* 49–52, May 8, 1989.

Goffman, Erving: *Relations in Public.* New York, Harper and Row, 1971.

Gold, John R.: Territoriality and human spatial behavior. *Progress in Human Geography, 6:* 44–67, 1982.

Haaland, Gordon: Economic determinants in ethnic processes. In Barth, Fredrik (ed.): *Ethnic Groups and Boundaries: The Social Organization of Cultural Difference.* London, George Allen and Unwin, 1969.

Hall, Edward Twitchell: *The Hidden Dimension.* Garden City, Doubleday, 1966.

Hall, Edward Twitchell: *The Silent Language.* New York, Fawcett, 1959.

Hartmann, Ernest: *Boundaries in the Mind: A New Psychology of Personality.* New York, Basic Books, 1991.

Healy, Bernadine: The Yentl syndrome. Editorial. *New England Journal of Medicine, 325:* 274–276, 1991.

Hinde, Robert Aubrey: *Biological Bases of Human Behavior.* New York, McGraw Hill, 1974.

Hirschhorn, Larry: *The Workplace Within: Psychodynamics of Organizational life.* Cambridge, MIT Press, 1988.

Holland, Agnieszka (Director); Menegoz, Margaret and Brauner, Arthur (Producers): *Europa, Europa* [Film]. France, Les Films Du Losange; Germany, CCC Filmkunst GMBH; Released by Orion Classics, 1990.

Johnson, Paul: *The Birth of the Modern: World Society 1815–1830.* New York: Harper Collins, 1991.

Jones, James H.: *Bad Blood: The Tuskegee Syphilis Experiment.* New York: Free Press, 1981.

Kanter, Rosabeth Moss: *The Change Masters.* New York, Simon and Schuster, 1983.

Kanter, Rosabeth Moss: Transcending business boundaries: 12,000 world managers view change. *Harvard Business Review, 69:* 151–164, May–June 1991.

Kee, Robert: *Ireland: A History.* Abacus edition. London, Sphere Books, 1982.

Knowles, Eric S.: Boundaries around social space: Dyadic responses to an invader. *Environment and Behavior, 4:* 437–445, 1972.

Kolers, Paul A.: Bilingualism and information processing. In Atkinson, Richard Chatham (ed.): *Contemporary Psychology.* San Francisco, W.H. Freeman, 1971.

Kuo, Zing Yang: Studies of the basic factors in animal fighting: VII. Interspecies coexistence in mammals. *Journal of Genetic Psychology, 97:* 211–225, 1960.

Lauderdale, Pat: Deviance and moral boundaries. *American Sociological Review, 41:* 660–676, 1976.

Leavitt, Judith Walzer: The medicalization of childbirth in the twentieth century. *Transactions and Studies of the College of Physicians of Philadelphia, 11:* 299–319, 1989.

Lyman, Stanford M. and Scott, Marvin B.: Territoriality: A neglected sociological dimension. *Social Problems, 15:* 236–249, 1967–1968.

Mahler, Margaret Schoenberger, Pine, Fred and Bergman, Anni: *The Psychological Birth of the Human Infant.* New York, Basic Books, 1975.

Marcos, Luis R., Urcuyo, Leonel, Kesselman, Martin and Alpert, Murray: The language barrier in evaluating Spanish-American patients. *Archives of General Psychiatry, 29:* 655–659, 1973.

Marden, Charles F.: *Minorities in American Society.* New York, American Book, 1952.

McCrone, John: *The Ape that Spoke: Language and the Evolution of the Human Mind.* New York, Morrow, 1991.

Mechanic, David: The growth of medical technology and bureaucracy: Implications for medical care. *Health and Society, Milbank Memorial Fund Quarterly, 55:* 61–78, 1977.

Milgram, Stanley: The experience of living in cities. *Science, 167:* 1461–1468, 1970.

Montagu, Ashley: *Touching: The Human Significance of the Skin.* New York, Columbia University Press, 1971.

Morgan, Kenneth O.: *The Oxford History of Britain.* Oxford, Oxford University Press, 1988.

Murphy, Jane M.: Psychiatric labeling in cross-cultural perspective. *Science, 191:* 1019–1028, 1976.

Nagi, Saad Z.: Teamwork in health care in the U.S.: A sociological perspective. *Milbank Memorial Fund Quarterly, 53:* 75–91, 1975.

Paris, Joel: Boundary and intimacy. *Journal of the American Academy of Psychoanalysis, 13:* 505–510, 1985.

Pliskin, Karen L.: *Silent Boundaries.* New Haven, Yale University Press, 1987.

Riffle, Kathryn L., Lamberth, Frances Hensailing, Moine, Gretchen L. and Fielding, Jane: Entry into practice: The continuing debate. In McCloskey, Joanne Comi and Grace, Helen Kennedy: *Current Issues in Nursing.* Second Edition. Boston, Blackwell, 1985.

Rivers, William Halse Rivers: *Psychology and Ethnology.* New York, Harcourt Brace, 1926.

Rivkin, Ellis: *The Shaping of Jewish History: A Radical New Interpretation.* New York, Scribner, 1971.

Rosenhan, D.L.: On being sane in insane places. *Science, 179:* 250–258, 1973.

Schaef, Anne Wilson and Fassel, Diane: *The Addictive Organization.* New York, Harper and Row, 1988.

Scott, Robert A.: *The Making of Blind Men.* New York, Russell Sage, 1969.

Shem, Samuel: *The House of God.* New York, Dell, 1978.

Sommer, Robert: *Personal Space: The Behavioral Basis of Design.* Englewood Cliffs, Prentice-Hall, 1969.

Sommer, Robert and Becker, Franklin D.: Room density and user satisfaction. *Environment and Behavior, 3:* 412–417, 1971.

Sontag, Susan: *Illness as a Metaphor.* New York, Farrar, Straus, and Giroux, 1978.

Starr, Paul: *The Social Transformation of American Medicine.* New York, Basic Books, 1982.

Stein, Jane J.: *Making Medical Choices: Who is Responsible?* Boston, Houghton Mifflin, 1978.

Stevens, Rosemary: *American Medicine and the Public Interest.* New Haven, Yale University Press, 1971.

U.S. Bureau of the Census: *Statistical Abstract of the United States: 1991.* 111 edition. Washington, U. S. Bureau of the Census, 1991.

Van Den Berghe, Pierre L.: Territorial behavior in a natural human group. *Social Science Information, 16:* 419–430, 1977.

Veness, Thelma: Introduction to hostility in small groups. In Carthy, John Dennis and Ebling, Francis John Govier (Eds.): *The Natural History of Aggression.* New York, Academic Press, 1964.

Wilber, Ken: *No Boundary.* Boston, New Science Library, 1981.

Wildavsky, Aaron Bernard: Doing better and feeling worse: The political pathology of health policy. In Knowles, John H. (ed.): *Doing Better and Feeling Worse: Health Policy in the United States.* New York, Norton, 1977.

Wilson, Edward Osborne: *Sociobiology: The New Synthesis.* London, Belknap Press, 1975.

Zerubavel, Eviatar: *The Fine Line: Making Distinctions in Everyday Life.* New York, Free Press, 1992.

Chapter 2

BOUNDARIES IN ORGANIZATIONS

The management of people is
the management of perceptions.

Charles E. Dwyer, Ph.D.
Wharton School of Business

Most organizations vacillate between highly permeable and impermeable boundaries, either of which present problems for an
organization. An organization with relatively impermeable boundaries
tends to be rigid and over controlled, while an organization with extremely
permeable boundaries is chaotic and disorganized. Alderfer (1976) refers
to the two extremes as "overbounded" and "underbounded" systems and
lists several characteristics that they share: (1) problems with authority;
(2) performance limited by role definitions; (3) problems in managing
human energy; (4) communication problems; and (5) confrontation with
certain life span issues—underbounded systems face issues of survival,
overbounded systems lose their ability to adapt (Alderfer, 1976). Boundary maintenance is essential in an organization because boundary problems result in ineffective task performance, conflict, and, eventually,
chaos.

Rice and his colleagues (1963, 1965) and Miller and Rice (1967) have
influenced our thinking about boundary function and control, the relationship between various parts of an organization to the total system, and
the dynamics of resistance to change. Rice assumes that each subgroup in
an organization gives voice to the unconscious tensions and anxieties
that are the collective legacy of the total organization. Problems in any
part of the system are felt in other parts of the system. As a result,
individuals and groups act to reduce tensions and restore equilibrium in
the organization (Klein and Gould, 1973).

Boundaries and boundary conflicts have numerous manifestations.
The following areas have been selected for discussion because they are
especially germane to managing boundaries in health organizations.

Types of Boundaries in Organizations

Economic

Reversing Alderfer's analysis, in which he listed boundary problems, we see a healthy system as one that makes maximum effective utilization of the people and resources in the system. By these criteria, our health care system has many dysfunctional features. Many of these arise from the economic basis of the system, particularly when government regulation provides one group with the power to aggregate to itself economic benefits desired by others. As we discussed in Chapter 1, governments can provide legal monopolies for health care professions by granting them the power to license on the grounds that they protect the population from charlatans. They also provide incentives for professionals to gain increased education to obtain increased income. The impulse to set educational standards and enforce them by licensure may, sometimes, be justifiable. For example, because the State of Texas puts few restraints on the activities of midwives, some low-income women and their children are at increased risk of birth complications and difficult deliveries.

State licensure is not the only path to monopoly and semimonopoly. Non-government boards and other such bodies can establish registration and certification policies that have the effect of law. For example, the American Society of Clinical Pathologists established an examination system and registration for medical technologists. It became the custom, in many laboratories, to hire only registered technologists. Their registration thus took on the form and effect of a license. Some states license medical technologists, but such licensure is far from universal. The clinical pathologists used their registration power to try to keep medical technologists from being employed by non-physician laboratory scientists. Before 1970, technologists who were employed by Ph.D. biochemists were threatened with the loss of their registration. An antitrust consent degree, signed by both the College of American Pathologists and the American Society of Medical Technologists, ended the threat of withdrawal of registration, but conflict regarding registration of medical technologists has been continuous (Brown, 1975), with both the American Society of Medical Technologists and the American Society of Clinical Pathologists registering medical technologists.

Health professions are not the only organized groups that seek State licensure or non-governmental certification to secure their economic position, but the health fields seem to be particularly subject to the pressures of economic conflict. Unlike retailers or service providers, such as roofers, barbers, etc., members of the health care professions provide services that cannot easily be evaluated by the consumer. The health care market does not seem to yield to the usual market pressures.

Economic pressures have resulted in savage competition between physicians and members of some outside groups, such as chiropractors. The American Medical Association tried to destroy the profession of chiropractic until it was forced to sign a consent decree by the antitrust division of the Department of Justice (Stolfi, 1979).

The monopoly enjoyed by the medical profession is not simply the result of government power. Starr (1982, p. 229) states:

> The triumph of the regular profession depended on belief rather than force, on its growing cultural authority rather than sheer power, on the success of its claims to competence and understanding rather than the strong arm of the police. To see the rise of the profession as coercive is to underestimate how deeply its authority penetrated the beliefs of ordinary people and how firmly it seized even the imagination of its rivals.

Nevertheless, the economic power afforded physicians by the restriction on hospital admissions and the prescription of drugs has caused conflicts among such diverse groups as clinical psychologists and psychiatrists, ophthalmologists and optometrists (Beachy, 1992). The outsider trying to understand these conflicts is unable to reach a balanced judgment because of the economic issues involved. As Starr notes, general practitioners within the medical profession resisted any attempts to grant specialists exclusive privileges over medical work. Thus, family physicians with limited training in mental health can prescribe powerful psychopharmacological drugs while clinical psychologists, who have had intensive training in mental health, cannot.

Starr has written at length about the attempts of the American medical profession to control its economic fate. By the 1990's, it had become apparent that attempts to provide universal health coverage with government programs, such as Medicare and Medicaid, resulted in enormous increases in health care costs, yet left millions of citizens with inadequate access to health care. Some type of cost control, with a concomitant control of health providers' incomes, seems inevitable, but the ultimate system, which may arise, remains unclear.

Economic concerns raise peculiar barriers to the evolution of an effective health care system. They also interfere, to a surprising degree, with the management of the system. For example, a bedside nurse may be the product of any one of at least four different educational levels: a one-year licensed practical (or vocational) nurse, an associate degree nurse, a three-year graduate of a hospital school of nursing, or a baccalaureate degree nurse (Cannings and Lazonic, 1975). Since the duties of nurses of different educational levels overlap, it is sometimes managerially difficult to adjust nursing duties to nursing education.

The linkage of pay, prestige, and assignment to educational level can interfere with the effective functioning of modern organizations, which generally try to base work assignments on demonstrated competencies. Preoccupation with education and certification overlooks the fact that much education is acquired on the job. Most American health care workers, by the time they've been working for five or ten years, have progressed far beyond the level of skills and abilities that they possessed upon initial registration, certification, or licensure.

Preoccupation with credentials clearly relates to the economic benefits of such credentials. The economic consequences to health care workers and institutions, such as hospitals, health professions schools, and insurance companies, will greatly influence the ways in which we finance and pay for health care.

Gender

Despite the increased number of women entering medicine, the legacy of centuries of gender bias continues to raise barriers to the effective functioning of the health care system. Denigrating the intelligence and capabilities of women, and labeling certain jobs as feminine and therefore less prestigious and desirable than others, has had serious effects on the functioning of hospitals, the recruitment of health care personnel, and the management of health care delivery. As the following statistics show, the system is largely staffed by females in low level positions and managed by males in prestigious roles. The situation is confounded by elitism since white males occupy most high level positions and minority females occupy most of the lowest level positions (Brown, 1975).

As Table 2-1 shows, modern American society employs many licensed and certified nurses, over 90% of whom are women. Data from the 1991 U.S. Census show that the number of women in medicine is growing rapidly, increasing from 15.8% in 1983 to 17.9% in 1989. Medical school enrollment data indicate that women will eventually comprise over one third of the total number of physicians. Comparable data for men in nursing show an increase from 4.2% to 5.8%. Thus, the number of women

TABLE 2-1
Number of Health Practitioners by Sex and Ethnicity

Occupation		Percent		
	Number	Female	Black	Hispanic
Diagnosticians				
Physicians	548, 000	17.9	3.3	5.4
Dentists	170, 000	8.6	4.3	2.9
Assessment and Treatment Personnel				
Registered Nurses	1, 599, 000	94.2	7.2	3.0
Pharmacists	174,000	32.3	4.7	2.2
Dieticians	83, 000	90.8	17.1	5.3
Inhalation Therapy	63, 000	52.5	12.5	2.7
Physical Therapy	90,000	77.3	4.8	6.1
Speech Therapy	63,000	88.6	3.3	0.9
Physician's Assistants	62,000	26.6	6.9	6.2
Health Technologists and Technicians				
Clinical Laboratory Technicians	308, 000	74.4	14.7	4.1
Dental Hygienists	80, 000	99.2	4.7	0.9
Health Record	72, 000	91.3	15.5	10.8
Radiologic Technicians	124, 000	75.8	10.1	4.3
Licensed Practical Nurses	414, 000	96.1	19.0	4.4
Health Service Personnel				
Dental Assistants	187, 000	98.9	7.4	9.0
Health Aides other than Nursing Aides	416, 000	84.5	17.7	7.0
Nursing Aides, Orderlies, and Attendants	1, 439, 000	90.4	31.4	6.0

Source: U.S. Bureau of the Census. *Statistical Abstract of the United States:1991.* 111th edition, Washington, D.C., U.S. Bureau of the Census 1991, pp. 395-397.

in medicine has increased, between 1983 and 1989, by 13%, while the number of men in nursing has increased by 38%. However, the number of women in nursing is so great that the identification of nursing as a female profession is apt to persist for many years. The data in Table 2-1 also reveal that employees in the health occupations are predominantly female, and that the least challenging of the health occupations generally employ the greatest number of minority personnel.

The virtual limitation of nursing to women does not mean that nursing is less challenging than medicine. Shryock (1959, p. 311) states that women nurses, by 1940, were doing more for patients than had physicians a half century earlier. The importance of gender in the health care occupations relates to the attitudes toward gender that have been held by society for years.

Several recent publications (e.g., Miller, 1986; Howell and Bayes, 1981) contain lengthy discussions of the influence of the tradition of male dominance and of fear of sexuality on the psychology of women. The influence of these traditions on the development of the largest health profession, nursing, is discussed by Shryock (1959). Shryock indicates that both medicine and nursing were undeveloped for most of recorded history. Modern nursing seems to have had its roots in the early middle ages:

> The actual care of hospital patients . . . was largely custodial in nature. It was provided . . . partly by monks or nuns and partly by servants. Just where the work of the religious stopped and that of servants began is difficult to say. The point is of some interest, since one of the difficulties in setting up the modern nursing profession was to disentangle it from a servant tradition (p. 110).

In Catholic countries, nursing was considered a religious vocation and was carried out mainly by nuns and monks. Male religious orders nursed in men's halls until the 19th century. Only male orderlies appeared in military hospitals until the 19th century. For three centuries following the Reformation, the nursing service in Protestant countries deteriorated (Shryock, 1959, pp. 160–168). Nursing became a woman's occupation, one plagued by poor pay, bad working conditions, confining discipline, and unattractive routine. The field was unattractive, except to those who could not get better jobs because of age, poverty, or ignorance. Unfortunately, early German attempts to select attendants more carefully were not very successful. Shryock (1959, pp. 235–236) suggests that superior women would not enter the service because domineering superintendents treated nurses as servants.

Medicine as a profession was plagued, for centuries, by a slavish adherence to ancient theories of illness. While scientific developments, in the 18th century, had great potential for influencing medicine, the vast majority of physicians were oblivious to these developments. It was not until the 19th century that modern medicine began to develop. The simultaneous recognition of the importance of nursing care led to the opening of the first nursing schools in the late 18th and early 19th centuries (Shryock, 1959, p. 235).

Florence Nightingale, whose work in England influenced nursing all over the world, changed the role of nursing and of women in nursing. Miss Nightingale received great publicity for her efforts to improve military medicine during the Crimean War between England and Russia. When she returned to England, she used her influence to establish nursing programs that followed two principles. First, she insisted on establishing independent nurse training institutions, thus preventing hospitals from exploiting nursing schools as cheap sources of personnel. Much of the subsequent history of the nursing and allied health professions revolves around attempts to transfer educational responsibilities from hospitals, which were viewed (often justifiably) as exploitative, to educational institutions. In the United States, hospitals, which did exploit their students, dominated nurse training. Second, Miss Nightingale insisted that nurses, rather than male hospital directors, whose treatment of nurses as servants caused low morale among nursing personnel, supervise nursing staff (Shryock, 1959, p. 279).

By the end of the 19th century, some male nurses still practiced in the military; however, the public generally regarded nursing to be a woman's vocation, probably because they thought women were more nurturing and sensitive than men.

Prevention vs. Rehabilitation

There is a sharp boundary between health and prevention and illness and rehabilitation and between mental and physical illness. Illness is the business of physicians, whereas health is everyone's responsibility. The reasons for much of the disability and death in the United States lie in the health practices and lifestyles of individuals. Since there is no known cure for many of our chronic diseases, future efforts must be directed toward preventing their occurrence. Educating patients about how to prevent disease and maintain their health is a major challenge to the health professions collectively and medicine specifically.

The failure of the medical profession to deal effectively with issues of health maintenance and prevention stems from the organizational structure of health care delivery and financing and the fact that procedure-oriented, high technology health care provides more prestige and higher incomes than does primary care (Colwill, 1992; Petersdorf, 1992). Specializing, for example, in the laser surgery of the eye results in greater economic rewards and prestige than practicing preventive medicine as a specialty or incorporating prevention into the treatment of the patient.

As George Bernard Shaw pointed out in his play, *The Doctor's Dilemma* (Shaw, 1957), physicians are mainly paid for treating illness, not for keeping patients healthy. Furthermore, health insurers pay most for dramatic treatments, such as surgery or diagnostic procedures, and very little for counseling or education, which may be the physician's main tools for preventive services. Often, insurance companies, in order to keep the cost of health insurance down, will not pay for routine preventive services, such as well baby checkups and, until recently, mammograms or pap smears. While public health officials, with some success, have been pressuring insurance companies to reimburse for preventive services, and recent legislation has promoted preventive services for indigent children and pregnant women, the neglect of simple preventive measures, such as immunizations, is a national scandal.

Specialization and subspecialization in the treatment of disease automatically exclude broad considerations of a person's whole body or general state of health. One consequence of physicians' tendency to focus on specific signs and symptoms of disease rather than address a patient's total condition is the frequent neglect of mental health. A significant number of patients suffer from depression, yet the diagnosis is often missed by primary care physicians (Eisenberg, 1992).

Kass (1975) points out that medicine must concern itself with health, not only with the cure of disease. Though medicine must remain, in large part, restorative and remedial, greater attention to healthy functioning and to regimens for becoming and remaining healthy could be salutary and help reduce the incidence of disease. Health is not a commodity to be delivered. Discovering what will promote and maintain health is only part of the challenge; we must also promote and inculcate good health habits and increase personal responsibility for health. One step in this direction is the public endorsement of the right to health. The right to health is unrealistic, given the fact that not every person has access to health care. Medical care is expensive and not equally available to all. Proposals for National Health Insurance simply make available to the uninsured what the privately insured now receive. As Kass points out, many of these proposals merely endorse current methods of providing medical care, but broaden the constituency. It is not only economic equality that is at issue. The health care system needs to be reoriented to pursue health, not just medical care. Proposals for National Health Insurance should try to embrace the importance of personal responsibility for health. They should contain incentives and provisions that would encourage healthy life styles, such as discounts for non-smokers and for people who attend classes or self-help groups to cut down or eliminate substance abuse and obesity.

In addressing the threats to health and to economic stability posed by unhealthy and dangerous life styles, we also should explore the unattractive aspects of our advertisement-drenched society. Cigarette smoking is glamorized by linking it to sports figures and heroic myths, such as the "Marlboro Man," and beer drinking is linked by commercials to fun and sexual pleasure. Athletics for youngsters should lead to life-long habits of physical exercise for all, not just glorify the athletic prowess of a few winners.

The boundaries between health and illness must change if we are to evolve an accessible, available, affordable system for preventing disease, minimizing disability, and maximizing people's total functioning. While most critics agree that prevention is good, they interpret the term in different ways. Disagreements are inevitable because they stem from two incompatible theories about the causes of illness in society (Taylor, 1982). Medical professionals debate the meaning and scope of preventive medicine. The field of preventive medicine is divided into three categories: tertiary prevention (the containment, amelioration, and cure of disease), secondary prevention (the detection and diagnosis of disease), and primary prevention (the removal of the underlying cause of disease through immunization, control of environmental factors, or modification of personal behavior). Historically, tertiary prevention has been the physician's proper domain. The debate widens when the proper method of primary prevention is addressed. Results from behavior modification are said to be small compared to those from state and federal actions against pollution and occupational hazards. Yet, it is argued that physicians need to try to modify the personal behavior of their patients (Taylor, 1982). In practice, physicians tend to focus on treatment to the detriment of prevention. When prevention is considered, the vaccine model of prevention dominates the physician's understanding of today's health problems (Eisenberg, 1977).

Mental vs. Physical Health

Especially neglected is the field of mental health. Much illness is directly related to stress, e.g., hypertension. Almost all illness is exacerbated by stress. Yet, the artificial boundaries between physical and mental health are further exacerbated, in the mental health field, by the different approaches of physicians and non-physicians. For example, non-psychiatric physicians may attempt to treat the organic symptoms caused by stress without dealing with the underlying emotional or environmental causes of the symptoms. If a patient visits a clinical psychologist or a psychiatric social worker for treatment of the symptoms of emotional illness, underlying physical causes, such as a tumor or a hormone imbalance, may be missed. A team approach may be the best way to deal with patient problems, but the boundaries that separate many health professions make it difficult to assemble effective teams.

A further danger to the effective functioning of society is the pressure created by dysfunctional organizations. Schaef and Fassel (1988) compare organizations to addictive individuals and point out that organizations, like individuals, can practice denial and dishonesty, isolation, self-centeredness, perfectionism, etc. Their metaphor may seem strained, yet organizational life, because of leaders who project their inadequacies upon other members of the organization, evidently can create unnecessary stress. Organizational stress probably contributes significantly to physical and emotional illness.

While the medical profession has asserted its authority in the field of prevention, it is not a pioneer. It cannot ignore the constituencies that support prevention and does not wish to watch a new, health-related area of activity grow and develop outside the domain of medicine. Rising medical care costs also pose problems for which competition and prevention have been viewed as solutions. The Carter Administration tried to expand both social and individualistic preventive measures, e.g., environmental curbs on industry, and attacks by health care agencies on unhealthy lifestyles. President Reagan's Administration continued efforts to prevent cancer through the National Cancer Institute's programs on the link between cancer and lifestyle, but curtailed social approaches to prevention, i.e., the hazardous waste program, air research, and the Centers for Disease Control budget.

The battle over prevention brings into conflict not only the interests of capital, labor, environmentalists, insurance companies, and the medical profession, but also those of government agencies, such as the Environmental Protection Agency, the Department of Health and Human Services, and the Office of Management and Budget. Some consensus that the public needs protection against pollution is emerging, leading to the passage, in 1991, of the Clean Air Act, which will force many painful choices on both business and consumers.

Other environmental threats to health are being ignored. Selcraig (1992) has documented the effects of cost reduction actions by chemical plants and years of neglect by the Occupational Safety and Health Administration (OSHA) on the safety of workers and citizens. As he points out, since 1986, there have been eighty-seven serious fires, leaks, and explosions in the oil-refining and chemical industries that have killed 159 people, injured at least 2,200 others, and caused more than $3 billion in property damage.

Because of the conflict between the need for health and safety and fear of the economic consequences of regulation, it has been difficult to reach a consensus on a strategy of prevention. Policy makers choose selectively from available research findings to justify their decisions about the strategies they choose to label prevention. In the immediate future, national policies probably will emphasize attacking self-destructive habits, although many problems that plague society are amenable to social action. Society chooses to ignore the social policy origins and possible solutions of many problems. For example, high school clinics that promote family planning can cut teenage pregnancies almost in half (Zabin et al., 1986, Edwards et al., 1977), yet arguments regarding the morality of birth control make it difficult to establish such clinics (Whitby, 1992). Policy makers persist in building additional prisons to handle the increase in drug-related crime without providing funds to treat the addicts who are imprisoned.

The individualist version of prevention makes sense to Americans, but, as preventive concerns attack their lifestyle and standard of living, the old boundaries between health and illness emerge. It is easier to turn ourselves over, when sick, to the miracles of medical technology than to inconvenience ourselves by altering the way in which we choose to live.

Political Boundaries

As Marmor *et al.* (1983) state, health is not a very useful category for political analysis. The health care industry is large and complex, and political battles range widely. Some programs influence the financing of care, others affect medical care resources, and still others affect regulation of personnel and programs. Controversy has focused on federal health programs and policies that affect everyone.

Throughout its history, the federal government has limited its health policies to crisis intervention and the control and prevention of disease in public health. Typically, federal intervention regarding health has been ad hoc, without an overall plan, formulation of objectives, or theoretical underpinning (Litman and Robins, 1984). National health policy has consisted of amorphous health goals with little coordination or follow-up. Many federal legislative initiatives, for the past several decades, have been idealistic, inconsistent, and, sometimes, contradictory.

The development of health policy began in 1910 with the Flexner report, which resulted in the closing of many medical schools and revitalization of the rest. Since then, despite the lack of a consistent health policy, health care has improved (Brown, 1978). The U.S. now spends more per capita than any other nation on health care, but ranks below the leading nations in quality of care as measured by mortality outcomes.

Health policy is rooted in the financial affairs relating to health. Health care is costly, and costs must be contained. Poor health is costly because it results in low productivity and lost wages and because the government must pay some form of insurance. A part of the problem in formulating health policy lies in the large number of players in the game (Brown, 1978). Decisions influencing financing or regulation create repercussions throughout the system. The fragmentation of the players is part of the difficulty in formulating a health policy. Physicians control almost 80 percent of the health dollars spent. The government pays 40 percent of the bills. Therefore, these groups have more influence than do consumers on the formulation of health care policy (Brown, 1978; Milio, 1981).

Milio (1981) asks, "What is the goal of health policy? Is its principal purpose to improve people's health or to provide them with personal health services?" If the primary goal of health policy is to improve health, we cannot continue to devote 86 percent of national health expenditures to the delivery of personal health services, which have limitations in promoting health. Programs should include ways to change working and living environments to make them more health-promoting. Health care policy must do more than make health services less costly (Milio, 1981). Our view of health must be broadened to go beyond the health of individuals or groups and encompass the total parameters of our society. As Blumstein and Zubkoff (1981) point out, "The issues must be dealt with in broad terms in recognition of the many components that enter into the production of good health."

Alford (1975, p. 249) has summarized the political and economic realities of health care and noted the barriers to structural change of health institutions as follows:

> The crisis of health care is *not* the result of the necessary competition of diverse interests, groups, and providers in a pluralistic and competitive health economy, nor is it a result of bureaucratic inefficiencies to be corrected by yet more layers of administration established by government policy. Rather, the conflicts between the professional monopolists who seek to erect barriers to protect their control over research, teaching, and care, and the corporate rationalizers who seek to extend their control over the organization of services . . . The integration of all aspects of health care — prevention, outpatient checkups, routine treatment for minor illnesses, specialized treatment for rare diseases or those requiring expensive machines, long-term care for chronic conditions — would require the defeat or consolidation of the social power that has been appropriated by various discrete interest groups and that preserves existing allocations of social values and resources.

Ginzberg (1990) has suggested that we will not reshape our national health policy unless we achieve consensus on key issues. We must be prepared to pay the cost of insuring access to health care for the entire population. Proposals that address only selected health issues are inadequate and insufficient; health system problems are interrelated. Proposals that seek to address one problem while exacerbating another are apt to be politically unstable and short-lived (Morone, 1990). The societal solutions to how we view health and how we provide health care are boundary issues. Conflicts between the boundaries and interests of providers and consumers have not yet caused a system breakdown, which will impel the parties to establish new boundaries that will yield an effective health system.

Elitism

As indicated earlier, white males hold most of the high prestige and high paying positions in the health care system, and black females hold most of the poorer paying, less prestigious jobs. Much of the elitism in the professions relates to the cost of professional education. The cost of tuition and deferred income required for professional education limits the ability of modest income families to provide such educational opportunities for their children. Because many medical students graduate with an enormous load of debt, it is difficult for them to pursue primary care positions when surgical and medical specialties are more lucrative. Health professions, which elevate educational standards and replace work study programs, like diploma schools of nursing, with college programs, limit opportunities for poor and disadvantaged young people who need to work while attending school. The closing of work study programs has also created shortages of health care personnel, and raised the salaries of those who can afford the education.

Since many minority members in American society are not only poor, but lack cultural values and traditions that emphasize education, the educated professions, for the most part, were closed to them until the 1970's, when the civil rights movement awakened society to inequities in the staffing of the professions. The number of Blacks and Hispanics entering the more prestigious health professions has now increased, but there is still a substantial gap between the proportion of these minority groups in the population and of those enrolled in health professions schools.

The social class gap between prestigious health professionals and the indigent is one reason for the neglect of the poor in our health care system. Few professionals from urban middle class areas care to practice in poor regions. In recent years, programs to recruit students from rural areas and expose them to rural medicine have had some success, but much remains to be done.

Inequities in the funding of health care have led many people to seek care at urban teaching hospitals where most physicians are trained. Patients depending upon exhausted residents in emergency rooms for their primary care often outnumber patients suffering from genuine medical emergencies. Therefore, residents and students often develop negative attitudes toward the urban poor who come to them for help (Shem, 1979). Users of emergency room facilities may suffer many indignities. Not only does the care they receive lack continuity and often ignore preventive medicine, the caregivers may be singularly unsympathetic.

Another species of elitism stems from the attitudes of most physicians toward primary care. Although the American public needs more primary care physicians and greater emphasis on health maintenance and preventive medicine, specialists have higher incomes and more prestige. Therefore, the number of students going into primary care has dropped (Colwill, 1992; Petersdorf, 1992). Overemphasis on high technology, tertiary health care creates boundaries against the development of an effective health care system.

Economic biases, gender biases, and ethnic biases reinforce snobbery and elitism. While public health workers and administrators, primary care providers, allied health professionals, nurses, and midwives provide many of the essential health care services that restore and maintain the health of most Americans, the greatest prestige goes to the highly paid, highly educated surgeons and specialists who use high technology.

Hierarchy in Organizations

The basic structure of all administrative systems is that of a pyramid. Occupying the apex of the pyramid is the chief executive. The next level contains the vice presidents in charge of finance, research, administration, sales, etc. The following level is that of middle management, which consists of the department heads operating within each division. Below management is the supervisory staff, members of which direct the workers who are at the base of the pyramid. The workers carry out direct services for the clients or customers, operate the machinery that produces the product, or do the actual physical work (Peter, 1986). Martin (1973), in his observations about various facets of "hierarchiology," enumerates several laws, among them: Martin's Law of Communication, "The inevitable result of improved and enlarged communication between different levels in a hierarchy is a vastly increased area of misunderstanding;" Hacker's Law of Personnel, "It is never clear just how many hands or minds are needed to carry out a process. Nevertheless, anyone having supervisory responsibility for the completion of a task will inevitably protest that his staff is too small for the assignment;" and Vail's Axiom, "In any human enterprise, work seeks out the lowest hierarchical level."

Today's health care system provides an excellent example of hierarchy; physicians are at or near the apex of the pyramid and paramedicals below. Furthermore, a hierarchy of prestige and authority exists among the paramedicals. Nurses, for example, are of higher status than attendants and technicians. The origins of this hierarchy are partly economic and partly class-related. Yet, in common with all hierarchies, the health care hierarchy developed, in large part, because it provided a fairly simple method of organizing large numbers of people to work together.

Each of us occupies a place in a number of pyramids—in our workplace, service and civic clubs, religious organizations, and families—and we all relate to the overall governmental pyramid that provides social organization for our society. Peter (1968) discussed the positive and negative aspects of this form of organization. On the negative side, layers of the pyramid can become obstacles to progress with minimal responsiveness to other layers of the bureaucracy, or a layer can become so involved in its own processes that it loses sight of the goals of the organization. On the positive side, various degrees of social organization take early discoveries to greater levels of usefulness and sophistication. Social and technological advances are interdependent.

Peter voiced the principle that systems start small and grow to occupy all of our time and space. In years past, Martin (1973) notes, everything was smaller and less complex, and the term, bureaucracy, was only applied to government. It specifically defined a method for the conduct of government business through a system of bureaus, or departments, each of which was under the control of a chief. Each bureau reported to a higher bureau chief, and so on, in a hierarchical form. A bureau chief's position in the hierarchy and the number of people over whom he or she had cognizance determined the bureau chief's prestige, power, and salary. The bureau system had built-in motivational pressures to: (1) increase the number of people in each bureau; (2) increase the number of bureaus; and (3) increase the number of levels in the hierarchy. Consequently, every element of the bureaucratic form of organization tended to promote organizational expansion.

The size and complexity of an organization or system must be appropriate to its function. As organizations or social institutions become larger and more complex, work becomes more specialized, and workers construct boundaries to protect their jobs. Managers also construct boundaries of varying permeability, to manage the workforce and to protect their turf.

When excessive bureaucratization creates problems for an organization because of the accumulation of dead wood, red tape, or any of the other symptoms of the Peter Pyramid Syndrome, analysis will reveal the need for ingenuity, innovation, and creativity. The creator is the innovator, the change agent, the problem solver. The conformist is the bureaucrat, the supervisor devoted to control and the achievement of measurable goals or products. Organizations need both types. However, the bureaucracy either forces creators out of the organization by requiring them to submit to boring, routine work, or continuously stifles their creativity so that they lapse into complacency (Peter, 1986). Creative persons are outnumbered by control-minded conformists; therefore, special efforts are needed to retain creative people in an organization. Organizations that have few, if any, creative people become rigid, focus on single issues, are reluctant to consider alternatives, and, as a result, become defensive. The boundaries of such organizations become battle stations that keep new ideas out and strengthen the hierarchy inside the organization. Such organizations become less responsive to their changing clients and the changing world in which the organization and clients live.

As Peter (1986) says, in our technological society, we often see new technology as the means of getting more work done in less time (e.g., E mail, computers, and FAX). However, new technology can increase the complexity of an organization or institution without improving its effectiveness. For example, all patient appointments in a large university hospital can be made by calling one number. If, however, the patient arrives at his appointment and finds inadequate and expensive parking facilities, waits several hours to see a health professional, and experiences rude treatment by personnel, the use of computers to improve health care access and quality has been of questionable value.

Peter (1986) proposes a total system perspective with the objective of doing more with less, "a simplified machine with no unnecessary parts." In total system management, managers have to be taught to deal with such intangibles as concepts, ideas, and values. Jobs become interlinked as employees minimize boundaries to meet client needs and attain the goals of the organization.

Boundary Personnel and Boundary Roles

Aldrich and Herker (1977) discuss the importance of boundary personnel in bringing innovation and change to an organization. They note that, by definition, all organizations have some boundary spanning roles, but some have an elaborate set of boundary roles while others have only a few. A small organization can survive with a simple structure, with few differentiated roles and functions. As organizational and environmental complexities increase, organizations can no longer afford nondifferentiated boundary spanning activities.

Thompson (1967) proposes three categories of boundary roles: mediating, long-linked, and intensive. Organizations with a mediating technology, like banks, insurance companies, federal express, or the postal service, hot lines, referral services, or information brokers, link clients with each other or with other organizations. Organizations in the book publishing and record producing industries that use a mediating technology were found to allocate many employees to boundary spanning roles. These boundary roles enable personnel to monitor the environment and provide information quickly to managers and executives.

Organizations with a long-linked technology, such as colleges, universities, and public schools, attempt to buffer most of their units and roles from the environment. They have few people in boundary roles. Since various organizational units are interdependent, there are many boundary roles between intra-organizational components. Long-linked technology gains maximum efficiency through standardized production of large volumes of output. Organizations employing long-linked technologies expand their domains vertically. Flawn (1990, pp. 22–23) describes the boundary spanning role of the president of a modern university as follows:

> The management of a large public university in the United States may well be the most difficult job in the world.... The president's problem is that by law, court decision, and board action, authority in universities has been cut into a number of pieces; the pieces have been parceled out to various constituencies; no single piece is big enough to permit action without consensus; there is never ready consensus about anything in universities.... But while the authority of university presidents is diminished, the responsibility that goes with the position is not. As a result, fewer and fewer presidents stay in the job very long.

Cohen and March (1986) describe a college president's job as one embracing "the ambiguities of anarchy." The authors conclude, "The contribution of a college president may often be measured by his capacity for sustaining that creative interaction of foolishness and rationality" (p. 229).

Organizations that use intensive technology also buffer most of their personnel from the environment. In intensive technology organizations concerned with people-changing activities, the client is temporarily assigned an organizational role and must change behavior to suit norms acceptable to the organization. Boundary personnel in this type of organization, e.g., the admitting physician in a hospital, the admissions officer at a private school, a police officer, or a judge, have the power to admit or reject clients. These organizations expand their domains by becoming "total institutions" and placing an impermeable boundary around their clients (Goffman, 1961). Aiken and Hage (1968) state that professionals in organizations engage in boundary-spanning contact to maintain contact with a professional reference group and keep abreast of changing technology in their fields.

Stable environments call for less monitoring than do unstable environments, and evoke fewer boundary roles. The film, record, book, and media industries provide examples of rapidly changing environments that require constant boundary spanning. Boundary roles in an organization become routinized to the degree that its leaders perceive a need to adapt to environmental change and to control the behavior of their workforce. Routinization can serve to maintain social control and limit the changing or sharing of boundary roles by employees. Boundary personnel in an organization can become powerful because they are information processors and negotiators with representatives outside the organization. They have a gatekeeper's power, and may become even more powerful if they make correct inferences and if their information is vital to the organization's survival (March and Simon, 1958). Boundary spanning people, however, spend a lot of time away from their organization, which often distances them from it (Allen and Seibert, 1990).

Two studies reported positive correlations between boundary spanning activity and job satisfaction (Keller and Holland, 1975; Keller, *et al.*, 1976). These studies also found small or insignificant correlations between role conflict, role ambiguity, and boundary spanning activity. Boundary spanning jobs permit persons to gain power, improve their bargaining position, increase their job satisfaction, and, perhaps, gain better jobs. Hierarchy is not inevitable; it is a manufactured need, one that can be reduced (Lawler, 1988). Organizations have reduced layers of management and staff groups to reduce costs only to have the levels of management reappear within a few years because no structural changes in the organization were made. If an organization is not redesigned, the need for a hierarchy will persist. Organizations that are designed to include work teams, new reward systems, extensive training, information systems, distribution of financial data, and the right kind of leader can function with less hierarchy.

Boundaries, Work Roles, and Work Satisfaction

Once managers understand the cultures of their organizations and have evaluated the environments, internal and external, they are ready to design a managerial control system. But first they must set the tone for their organizations. The style and philosophy of management affect the culture of an organization. Organization and corporate culture consists of the shared values, perceptions, and goals that members of an organization apply to its activities and problems (Asay and Maciariello, 1991). Thomas Watson, the founder of IBM, attributed his company's success primarily to the power of beliefs. These beliefs, which also could be the foundation for any medical organization, include respect for the individual, customer service, and dedication to excellence.

A manager gets things done by delegating tasks. The manager must be a catalyst. Management style is most effective when it is flexible. While managers' styles may differ and still attain the same organizational goals, the most effective managers use whichever style is most appropriate at the time and for the individual. Managing people is a process. Too often, in the workplace, workers perceive an impermeable boundary between their job and opportunities to grow and advance. Management often conveys the message that workers who are eager to learn new skills are only interested in enhancing their advancement within or without the organization. Management often perceives workers who express the desire to learn and to grow as disloyal.

Good personnel managers see the mission of the workplace as a transaction between the values of the employees and the values of the organization. Managers can encourage employees to do their jobs, or managers can encourage employees to find innovative ways to do their jobs better and to acquire new skills. Managers must be in touch with the values of their employees, as well as aware of their own values, if the workplace is to be mutually satisfying and productive. The personal values of the manager have a major impact on the treatment of employees. Managers who view profit maximization as an important goal will be less willing to spend money on improving cafeteria and restroom facilities than will managers for whom compassion is an important value. Value patterns are predictive of success and could be used in selection and placement decisions. There are some disadvantages in having employees and managers with value profiles that are too much alike. A mix of values is, perhaps, more conducive to maintaining organizational vitality and adaptation to changing needs.

Karasek and Theorell (1990) point out that the productivity problems of work require the same solutions that enhance employee health. Low-decision-latitude jobs carry the highest risk of heart disease, and also waste employee skills. They speculate that much more desirable jobs could be designed by avoiding low levels of decision latitude, in which increasing output demands result in increased stress and even heart disease, but no increase in productivity. If jobs could be redesigned with high decision latitude—opportunities for taking responsibility through participative decision-making—demands would be seen as challenges and would be associated with increased learning and motivation, more effective performance, and less risk of illness.

John Ruskin said, "In order that people may be happy in their work, these three things are needed: They must be fit for it, they must not do too much of it, and they must have a sense of success in it." Data from several studies of stress, social support, and health consistently support the proposition that social support can reduce work stress, improve health, and lessen the impact of work stress on health. A healthy workplace is one in which management recognizes the need for social support and tries to find ways to meet the need for employees at all levels of the organization. In the workplace, many sources of stress can be identified, altered, or reduced to enhance the productivity and efficiency of the total organization (Bruhn and Cordova, 1987).

Work as a job and work as a career are opposite ways of viewing work. There is, however, a common element in both—job satisfaction. The degree of congruence between individual work values and what the job delivers results in some level of job satisfaction. Job satisfaction directly affects work attitudes. As several authors point out, people "actualize" their potentials and capacities through work. A significant source of job stress is created when self-actualization at work is thwarted and work becomes a necessity, routine, and unsatisfying (Bruhn, 1989).

If the boundaries between work values and employee values are fixed and rigid, managers are likely to see employee dissatisfaction, low morale, and continual turnover. Placement in a job is not a one-time action for an employer. Continuous feedback regarding expectations and performance should occur, throughout employment, between the employer and employee. People need to know where they stand with respect to their performance. Individuals differ in the criteria they use to assess how well they are doing. People who are unsure about their abilities or personal attributes can have problems in developing appropriate levels of aspiration or understanding their competence for certain tasks; these people can be the proverbial square pegs. They may be unable to do the job; the job may be beneath or beyond their capacities. Such people will, eventually, experience some form of social punishment at every turn. The anticipation of such consequences is sufficient to generate stress (Bruhn, 1979).

Training for specific jobs can lead to what has been called the permanence fallacy or final placement syndrome. If employees like their work, perform satisfactorily, and have favorable evaluations from their supervisors, employers may envision them in their jobs permanently. Furthermore, the employees are happy. To move those employees would mean finding and training replacements who might not perform as well. How well employees fit their jobs, adjust to their jobs, and like their jobs are all facets of a complicated phenomenon called job satisfaction. Job satisfaction can change, so any assessment of it must be timebound (Bruhn, 1979).

Argyris (1957) believes that our society sees the work situation as a place to be productive, and the worker as a machine whose job is to produce. Tasks are sterile and limited. Little, if anything, is expected of the worker besides performance of his specific job. To dramatize these points, he brought mental patients into a factory to do routine jobs. The patients increased production by 400 percent. They were easy to supervise and worked without complaint. While robot workers could increase production, Argyris believes that it is important to consider the whole person and to treat workers as adults; production and economic incentives are often stressed more than the human side of the workplace.

In a study of attitudes toward work, researchers interviewed 200 engineers and accountants, representing a cross section of Pittsburgh industry, about events they experienced at work that resulted in either a notable improvement or a significant reduction in job satisfaction (Herzberg, 1966). Five strong factors in determining job satisfaction—achievement, recognition, work itself, responsibility, and advancement—stood out, the last three having greater importance for lasting attitude change. These five factors, called motivators, were seldom mentioned when the respondents spoke of job dissatisfaction.

Managers should gear their activities to the employees' levels of maturity with the overall goals of helping them to develop as persons, to require less external control, and to gain more self-control (Hersey and Blanchard, 1972). One reason people change jobs is that they are not happy. They may be unhappy at work because they are unhappy in other life roles, or because their life away from work prevents them from gaining satisfaction from their jobs. Finding, selecting, placing, training, and retaining workers is a highly individualistic process. Our society puts a high value on work, and we spend most of our lives working. It is important that this time be meaningful and satisfying to the individual and productive for the organization.

Davis (1975) points out the existence of a law of diminishing returns in organizational behavior. This law warns management that, although increased worker autonomy, employee security, or employee specialization can be beneficial, in excess, they will be counterproductive. The law of diminishing returns applies to all levels of an organization, including management; for any situation, a desirable practice can surpass the point at which it is most effective.

Karasek and Theorell (1990) review the literature on organizational restructuring to build "learning-based" organizations: organizations that replace fixed form, hierarchical bureaucracies with flexible structures, which can adapt to changing external conditions and changing employee capabilities. It is their premise that learning occurs more easily under circumstances in which decision latitude is commensurate with the challenge, not overwhelmed by it, as in crisis-learning situations. One new perspective in organizational change literature is that of change-process democracy, the empowerment of lower-level employees. Consultants and managers, in this perspective, help employees to find their own solutions through problem analysis and trial and error. Employees develop their own models of the work process instead of uncritically adopting a cookbook prescription from management. Karasek and Theorell (1990) propose that the technical and social systems of work need to be reorganized together. They propose lifting the boundaries between the technological and human sides of work and between preserving environmental harmony with management and promoting the job satisfaction of individual workers. They propose developing a work environment that would focus not only on output, but also on developing the creative skills and capabilities of the workers. This could have positive benefits, not only for the organization, but for society as a whole.

Those acquainted with health care facilities are aware of obstacles to the ideals regarding personnel management. The fragmentation of health care personnel into dozens of specialized occupations and levels makes it difficult to assign employees to meaningful roles that are developed on the job. While the specialized nature of the required job skills, such as those needed to operate complex machinery, makes formal training essential, fragmentation into specialties can make work reassignments difficult. Middle-aged medical technologists find today's laboratories vastly different from those of the past, yet they have learned how to operate complex machinery while retaining their roles as laboratory specialists. While it may be possible to train radiological technicians to run automated chemistry equipment in a brief period of time, such an action would not benefit the radiological technicians; they could not be certified to perform such tasks without fulfilling new educational requirements. Such an approach may not be feasible because of the need for special technical school training, but industry routinely carries out such job reassignments. In many organizations, a secretary can advance to levels of management, especially if training opportunities are made available to supplement on-the-job experience. The rigid job classifications in the health care system make such moves extremely difficult.

Another problem in many health care facilities is the use of vertical management structures, which inhibit the ability of management to deal with problems on site. Because nurses believed that male physicians would not pay proper attention to nurses' abilities and skills, and because of professional suspicion that only one member of a profession can supervise another, health care facilities use a dual management structure. Physicians might find one or more nurses in their clinics to be inadequate, but they have no direct supervision of the nurses. The physician with personnel problems must deal with the Director of Nursing Services (Brown and Henry, 1987, Haimann, 1973, pp. 103–104).

A positive development in medical care has been the creation of multi-disciplinary patient care teams, such as those that have been organized to manage children born with a cleft lip or palate. A child born with a cleft palate or split lip requires the cooperative care of plastic surgeons, dentists, pediatricians, social workers, psychologists, otolaryngologists, speech pathologists, audiologists and team coordinators (Kaufman, 1991). The cleft palate team at the University of Texas Medical Branch at Galveston, over many years, has enrolled over 300 patients, and has succeeded in helping them overcome multiple problems and lead almost normal lives. Multidisciplinary teams, bound by a common desire to help severely ill patients, develop strong bonds of mutual respect. Such teams have been developed to care for burn and trauma patients, elderly patients, patients suffering from child abuse, etc. Hopefully, the model of the cooperative team may eventually replace the model of the hierarchical organizational structure, which focuses principally on the directors of the hierarchy.

Boundaries and Professional Autonomy

A major reason for forming organizations is their ability to accomplish things that individuals cannot. An individual may become a great solo pianist, but the symphony orchestra provides us with an additional world of music. Such an organization does not simply produce more music more efficiently than the individual pianist; it produces a *kind* of music that could not be produced by an individual or by any number of unorganized individuals. Similarly, a surgeon cannot perform surgery efficiently or safely without the assistance of the anesthesiologist, nurses, residents, and other technicians.

While organization plays an important role, it must be seen in perspective with culture. For example, it is not only because of the organization of hospitals, training of nurse midwives, and improved technology that we have been able to reduce infant mortality rates. A better educated public has helped by participating in improved prenatal and postnatal care. Similarly, the successes in the exploration of space depend as much on developments in culture as they do on advances in technology.

Organizations derive functions, such as the education of children, the production of cars, the distribution of news, or the maintenance of health, from the society in which they exist. Because these functions are diverse and complex, a system for subdividing tasks allocates them to groups or individuals with the appropriate skills, and coordinates their activities. This style of organization is called bureaucracy. Bureaucracy has several characteristics: (1) the division of labor is clear cut, each task is performed by a specialist; (2) in a clear hierarchy of administrative authority, each official has authority over his subordinates, but is accountable to his superiors for the subordinates' actions; (3) explicit rules are designed to assure uniformity of performance in accord with role prescriptions; (4) a detached, impersonal approach is taken in all matters; and (5) technical qualifications determine the assignment of personnel to each role. Bureaucratic organization is designed to maximize rationality in the performance of complicated tasks.

In the health care bureaucracy, the physician occupies the key role in the division of labor. In virtually every case, the physician is nominally in control, whether in solo fee-for-service practice or as chief of service in a large hospital employing many other health professionals (Rosengren, 1980). A central feature of this authority is the physician's general capacity to influence others in providing health care. The physician is professionally and organizationally mandated to initiate actions and to direct others to carry them out. He or she is a manager, programmer, and coordinator for the division of labor in health care, with the exception, in certain circumstances, of such health professionals as nurses, occupational therapists, and physical therapists, and others who are permitted by law to engage in independent practice. However, the members of various health professional groups are continually maneuvering and negotiating for more authority, power, and status (Rosengren, 1980). Professional status parallels a group's distinctive decision-making prerogatives. Given the distribution of rights, obligations, and authority within the health professions, a complex of stress and conflict is highly likely.

A major variable affecting relationships among health occupations is autonomy, the degree to which members of an occupation can work independently of medical supervision and the degree to which they can attract their own clientele. On the whole, the more autonomous the occupation, the greater is the potential for conflict. Few of the present paramedical occupations deal with autonomous areas.

Freidson (1970) points out another factor that distinguishes among the health occupations, professionalism. Professionalism is a set of attributes that is characteristic of professionals, such as commitment to one's work as a career and an emphasis on public service rather than private profit. It has not been established that professionalism distinguishes the occupations in the division of labor. Professionalism seems to exist independently of professional status. Paramedical occupations, which are dominated by medicine, are often considered "less professional" because of differences in training, scope of work, and so forth. A profession is distinct from other occupations in that its members have the right to control their own work, but workers in other occupations are not necessarily less professional in the way they work.

Karasek and Theorell (1990) suggest that sharing decision-making powers among health care disciplines could yield more productivity and job satisfaction, but the granting of such rights is often resisted because it involves crossing boundaries created by professional education and training. Some higher-level professionals were unwilling to share responsibilities with competent lower-level professionals because the higher-level professionals had made a large investment in educational training and wanted both economic and career development rewards from that investment (Karasek and Theorell, 1990). Resistance to yielding jealously guarded boundaries is the major obstacle to reallocating role responsibilities. However, this hurdle is grounded in social traditions, not policy, and, therefore, is subject to change.

Technology is forcing many occupations to cross boundaries. Karasek and Theorell (1990) propose the despecialization of society as a whole through job redesign—not a total rejection of specialization, but a return from current levels of fragmentation. Work roles in Japan are worth examining (Ouchi, 1981). The Japanese emphasize lifetime rotation through many roles, nonspecialized career paths, holistic problem analysis, and consensus-building. Productivity is a problem of managerial organization. Trust and a sense of communal responsibility are the essential ingredients of Ouchi's Theory Z. In the U.S., we have become too narrowly focused in looking at our health care system, seeking economic and political answers to basic questions regarding the value of health and the quality of life. Perhaps, we must commit ourselves to a common health care goal rather than allow our society's need for an effective health care system to be secondary to individual desires for power, prestige, and economic reward. This would require boundary modifications beyond those that we have considered to date.

Technological Innovation and Boundaries

Almost every technological advance affects health and human disease and consequently affects medical practice. Medical innovations directly and intimately influence whether and how we live and when and how we die (Dutton, 1988). For example, development of improved techniques to prevent conception resulted in a reduction in the birth rate. This led to a reduction in the demand for food and an increase in parents' ability to provide children with educational opportunities. Negative consequences of contraceptives include the increased risk of thrombotic disease, the yet unproven suspicion of liver disease or certain forms of cancer from "the pill," and the guilt associated with preventing conception in members of some religious groups (Sidel, 1971).

All technological advances have a paradoxical relationship to the human condition. Practical problems—moral, legal, social, economic, and political—derive from new biomedical technologies, for example: the legality and morality of abortion, the definition of clinical death, the legitimacy of research on fetuses, the morality of test-tube babies and surrogate motherhood, the propriety of sperm banks, the right to refuse medical treatment, the rationale for psychosurgery, the just distribution of medical resources, the dangers and benefits of gene splicing, and the use and abuse of psychoactive drugs (Kass, 1985).

Humanity may consciously modify the nature of the human species and control its behavior. Manipulation of genetic material, perfection of methods for long-term contraception, controlled fertilization, and application of eugenics principles could lead to control of all human reproductive processes. To achieve given social goals, society might limit the right to procreate to those with the most favorable genes. The reproductive function could be separated from marriage, and even from the family (Pellegrino, 1971). Innovations in biomedical science and technology create the need for methods of social regulation and control, which could range from self regulation by physicians and scientists to formal governmental controls (Mendelsohn, et al., 1971).

The introduction of new and expensive products of medical technology is, at least in part, to blame for rising medical costs (Caplan, 1986). Comroe and Dripps (1976) have provided a partial list of products of medical technology introduced since 1950: automated blood chemistries, ultrasound, CAT scan, NMR scan, artificial organs, pacemakers, angioplasty, laser surgery, organ transplants, intracardiac surgery, anticoagulants, cortical implants, oral diuretics, parenteral nutrition, intensive care, fiberoptic catheters, and a host of vaccines and drugs. These innovations have raised several issues, including the rationing of certain types of care, known as the "no fat" thesis of technology, and the need for adequate assessment and control of existing and evolving medical technology. Some ethicists are concerned about how "we can learn how to institutionalize 'playing God' while still maintaining the key elements of a free society" (McDermott, 1967). Trosko (1984) has described the "Pontius Pilate syndrome," which, he says, is a characteristic feature of technological intervention in Western culture. He points out that we too often intervene with technology and wash our hands of its long-term consequences. We find cultural and moral support for putting the plug in, but find little support for the consequences of having to pull it out.

Schwitalla (April 1929) stated,

> Research is a bugbear to some people; a shibboleth to others. Some have found it to be an incubus; others have found it the guiding torch of truth. Some regard it as a gift of the gods; others find it the millstone on the neck of progress ... and yet the fact is definite and clear, simple, and unmistakable, that research among all human agencies has been the outstanding factor in the material development of our civilization.

No one wants to return to the medical system of the past with its staggering toll of babies and young children lost to epidemics and infant diarrhea, mothers lost in childbirth, promising young people, like John Keats, lost to tuberculosis and other diseases that, today, are relatively rare, and the warehousing, for decades, of people suffering from psychoses. The roles of physicians have been affected greatly by the availability of advanced technologies for diagnosis and treatment. The doctor-patient relationship has been diluted by shuttling patients to different health services. The diversification of technology has fragmented patient care. It is said that thirteen health care workers support each physician (Rushmer, 1980). Advances in some technologies—for example, imaging technology, nuclear magnetic resonance, digital subtraction angiography, diagnostic ultrasound, computerized tomography, and photo emission tomography—have created new specialties among the allied health disciplines. Each new technology requires a new vocabulary and skills. The creation of new disciplines and subspecialties will create new boundaries among existing disciplines (Bruhn and Philips, 1985), and increase the need to overcome these boundaries by organizing therapeutic teams.

Although much of the new technology, such as the development of radiology, has clear and obvious benefits, newer technology is often seen as an overrefinement of existing methods. Does open heart surgery really improve the quality of life over pharmacologic methods of handling coronary heart disease (Jenkins et al., 1983)? Much of the controversy concerning technology relates to questions about whether any new product, service, or process represents an improvement or a liability. Resolution of this dispute will not be simple. Any technological innovation has costs and benefits. Any solution will be dependent on the balance between these two and on whomever is doing the balancing (Bennett, 1977).

REFERENCES

Aiken, Michael and Hage, Jerald: Organizational interdependence and intra-organizational structure. *American Sociological Review, 33:* 912–930, 1968.

Alderfer, Clayton P.: Boundary relations and organizational diagnosis. In Meltzer, Hyman and Wickert, Frederic R. (eds.): *Humanizing Organizational Behavior.* Springfield, IL, Charles C Thomas, 1976.

Aldrich, Howard and Herker, Diane: Boundary spanning roles and organization structure. *The Academy of Management Review, 2:* 217–230, 1977.

Alford, Robert R.: *Health Care Politics.* Chicago, University of Chicago Press, 1975.

Allen, Myria Watkins and Seibert, Joy Hart: Communicators spanning the boundaries: A story of power, loyalties, and stress. In Sypher, Beverly Davenport (ed.): *Case Studies in Organizational Communication.* New York, Guilford, 1990.

Argyris, Chris: *Personality and Organization: The Conflict Between System and the Individual.* New York, Harper, 1957.

Asay, Lyal D. and Maciariello, Joseph A.: *Executive Leadership in Health Care.* San Francisco, Jossey-Bass, 1991.

Beachy, Debra: Doctors defend their turf: Rivals expanding job descriptions. *Houston Chronicle, 91:* 1F, 5F, March 22, 1992.

Bennett, Ivan L., Jr.: Technology as a shaping force. In Knowles, John F. (ed.): *Doing Better and Feeling Worse: Health in the United States.* New York, Norton, 1977.

Blumstein, James F. and Zubkoff, Michael: In McKinlay, John B. (ed.): *Politics and Health Care.* Cambridge, MIT Press, 1981.

Brown, Carol A.: Women workers in the health service industry. *International Journal of Health Services, 5:* 173–184, 1975.

Brown, Barbara and Henry, Beverly: Nursing education administration, practice, and research. In Wolper, Lawrence F. and Penna, Jesus J. (eds.): *Health Care Administration: Principles and Practices.* Rockville, Aspen, 1987.

Brown, Jack Harold Upton: *The Politics of Health Care.* Cambridge, Ballinger, 1978.

Bruhn, John G.: Job stress: An opportunity for professional growth. *Career Development Quarterly, 37:* 306–315, 1989.

Bruhn, John G.: Square pegs and round holes: Job satisfaction and the health of workers. *Health Values, 3:* 310–315, 1979.

Bruhn, John G. and Cordova, F. David: Promoting healthy behavior in the workplace. *Health Values, 11:* 39–48, 1987.

Bruhn, John G. and Philips, Billy U.: The influence of technology on the future of allied health professionals. *Journal of Allied Health, 14:* 289–295, 1985.

Cannings, Kathleen and Lazonick, William: The development of the nursing labor force in the United States: A basic analysis. *International Journal of Health Services, 5:* 185–216, 1975.

Caplan, Arthur L.: The high cost of technological development: A caveat for policymakers. In Allen, Anne S. (ed.): *New Options, New Dilemmas.* Lexington, D.C. Heath, 1986.

Cohen, Michael D. and March, James G.: *Leadership and Ambiguity.* 2nd ed. Boston, Harvard Business School Press, 1986.

Colwill, Jack M.: Where have all the primary care applicants gone? *New England Journal of Medicine, 326:* 387–383, 1992.

Comroe, Julius H., Jr. and Dripps, Robert D.: Scientific basis for support of biomedical science. *Science, 192:* 105–108, 1976.

Davis, Keith: A law of diminishing returns in organizational behavior. *Personnel Journal, 54:* 616–619, 1975.

Dutton, Diana Barbara: *Worse than the Disease: Pitfalls of Medical Progress.* Cambridge, Cambridge University Press, 1988.

Edwards, Laura E., Steinman, Mary E., Hakanson, Erick Y.: An experimental comprehensive high school clinic. *American Journal of Public Health, 67:* 765–766, 1977.

Eisenberg, Leon: Treating depression and anxiety in primary care: Closing the gap between knowledge and practice. *New England Journal of Medicine, 326:* 1080–1083, 1992.

Eisenberg, Leon: The perils of prevention: A cautionary note. Editorial. *New England Journal of Medicine, 297:* 1230–1232, 1977.

Flawn, Peter Tyrell: *A Primer for University Presidents: Managing the Modern University.* Austin, University of Texas Press, 1990.

Freidson, Eliot: *Profession of Medicine.* New York, Dodd, Mead, 1970.

Ginzberg, Eli: *The Medical Triangle: Physicians, Politicians, and the Public.* Cambridge, Harvard University Press, 1990.

Goffman, Erving: On the characteristics of total institutions. In Cressey, Donald Ray (ed.): *The Prison: Studies in Institutional Organization and Change.* New York, Holt, Rinehart, and Winston, 1961.

Haimann, Theo: *Supervisory Management for Health Care Institutions.* St. Louis, Catholic Hospital Association, 1973.

Hersey, Paul and Blanchard, Kenneth H.: *Management of Organizational Behavior Utilizing Human Resources.* 2nd ed., Englewood Cliffs, Prentice-Hall, 1972.

Herzberg, Frederick: *Work and the Nature of Man.* New York, World, 1966.

Howell, Elizabeth and Bayes, Marjorie (eds.): *Women and Mental Health.* New York, Basic Books, 1981.

Jenkins, C. David, Stanton, Barbara Ann, Savageau, Judith A., et al.: Coronary artery bypass surgery: Physical, psychological, social, and economic outcomes six months later. *JAMA, 250:* 782–788, 1983.

Karasek, Robert and Theorell, Töres: *Healthy Work: Stress, Productivity, and the Reconstruction of Working Life.* New York, Basic Books, 1990.

Kass, Leon R.: Regarding the end of medicine and the pursuit of health. *The Public Interest, 40:* 11–42, 1975.

Kass, Leon R.: *Toward a More Natural Science.* New York, Free Press, 1985.

Kaufman, Felix: Managing the cleft lip and palate patient. *Pediatric Clinics of North America, 38:* 1127–1147, 1991.

Keller, Robert T. and Holland, Winford E.: Boundary-spanning roles in a research and development organization: An empirical investigation. *Academy of Management Journal, 18:* 388–393, 1975.

Keller, Robert T., Szilagyi, Andrew D., and Holland, Winford E.: Boundary-spanning activity and employee reactions: An empirical study. *Human Relations, 29:* 699–710, 1976.

Klein, Edward B. and Gould, L.J.: Boundary issues and organizational dynamics: A case study. *Social Psychiatry, 8:* 204–211, 1973.

Lawler, Edward E., III: Substitutes for hierarchy. *Organizational Dynamics, 17:* 5–15, 1988.

Litman, Theodor J. and Robins, Leonard S.: *Health Politics and Policy.* New York, Wiley, 1984.

March, James G. and Simon, H.: *Organizations.* New York, Wiley, 1958.

Marmor, Theodore R., Dunham, Andrew, and Greenberg, Julie: The politics of health. In Mechanic, David (ed.): *Handbook of Health, Health Care, and the Health Professions.* New York, Free Press, 1983.

Martin, Thomas Lyle, Jr.: *Malice in Blunderland.* New York, McGraw-Hill, 1973.

McDermott, Walsh: Opening comments: A colloquium on ethical dilemmas from medical advances. *Annals of Internal Medicine, 67(3, Part II):* 39–42, 1967.

Mendelsohn, Everett, Swazey, Judith, and Taviss, Irene (eds.): *Human Aspects of Biomedical Innovation.* Cambridge, Harvard University Press, 1971.

Milio, Nancy: *Promoting Health through Public Policy.* Philadelphia, F.A. Davis, 1981.

Miller, Eric John and Rice, Albert Kenneth: *Systems of Organization.* London, Tavistock, 1967.

Miller, Jean Baker: *Toward a New Psychology of Women.* 2nd edition. Boston, Beacon, 1986.

Morone, James A.: Beyond the words: The politics of health care reform. *Bulletin of the New York Academy of Medicine, 66:* 344–365, 1990.

Ouchi, William G.: *Theory Z.* New York, Avon, 1981.

Pellegrino, Edmund D.: Physician, patients, and society: Some new tensions in medical ethics. In: Mendelsohn, Everett, Swazey, Judith, and Taviss, Irene (eds.): *Human Aspects of Biomedical Innovation.* Cambridge, Harvard University Press, 1971.

Peter, Laurence J.: *The Peter Pyramid.* New York, Morrow, 1986.

Petersdorf, Robert G.: Primary care applicants—they get no respect. *New England Journal of Medicine, 326:* 408–409, 1992.

Rice, Albert Kenneth: *Learning for Leadership.* London, Tavistock, 1965.

Rice, Albert Kenneth: *The Enterprise and its Environment.* London, Tavistock, 1963.

Rosengren, William R.: *Sociology of Medicine: Diversity, Conflict, and Change.* New York, Harper and Row, 1980.

Rushmer, Robert Frazer: *National Priorities for Health: Past, Present, and Projected.* New York, Wiley, 1980.

Schaef, Anne Wilson, Fassel, Diane: *The Addictive Organization.* New York, Harper & Row, 1988.

Schwitalla, Alphonse M.: The real meaning of research and why it should be encouraged. *Modern Hospital, 32(4):* 77–80, 1929.

Selcraig, Bruce: Bad chemistry: How Reaganomics has fueled Texas plant explosions. *Harper's, 284:* 62–73, April 1992.

Shaw, George Bernard: The doctor's dilemma. In: *Selected Plays of Bernard Shaw.* Vol. 1. New York, Dodd Mead, 1957.

Shem, Samuel: *The House of God.* New York, Dell, 1978.

Shryock, Richard Harrison: *The History of Nursing: An Interpretation of the Social and Medical Factors Involved.* Philadelphia, Saunders, 1959.

Sidel, Victor W.: New technologies and the practice of medicine. In Mendelsohn, Everett, Swazey, Judith, and Taviss, Irene (eds.): *Human Aspects of Biomedical Innovation.* Cambridge, Harvard University Press, 1971.

Starr, Paul: *The Social Transformation of American Medicine.* New York, Basic Books, 1982.

Stolfi, Julius E.: AMA surrenders to chiropractors. *New York State Journal of Medicine, 79:* 782–787, 1979.

Taylor, Rosemary C.R.: The politics of prevention. *Social Policy, 13:* 32–41, 1982.

Thompson, James D.: *Organizations in Action.* New York, McGraw-Hill, 1967.

Trosko, James E.: Scientific views of human nature: Implications for the ethics of technological intervention. In Brock, D. Heyward (ed.): *The Culture of Biomedicine: Studies in Science and Culture.* Vol. 1. Cranbury, Associated University Presses, 1984.

U.S. Bureau of the Census. *Statistical Abstract of the United States: 1991.* 111th edition. Washington, U.S. Bureau of the Census, 1991.

Whitby, Bob: Clergy says condom plan plain wrong. *Galveston Daily News, 149:* 1A, April 5, 1992.

Zabin, Laurie S., Hirsch, Marilyn B., Smith, Edward A., et al.: Evaluation of a pregnancy program for urban teenagers. *Family Planning Perspectives, 18:* 119–126, 1986.

Chapter 3

BOUNDARY ISSUES IN
THE HEALTH PROFESSIONS

Its the job of a chief executive to see around corners. And
the stark fact is, I didn't see around this one.

Donald Kennedy, 1991
President
Stanford University

Professional autonomy is buttressed by the tendency toward territoriality that is typical of most humans and is also reinforced by the rituals and educational traditions of the professions. In his book, *Doctors*, Segal points out the boundaries that separate medicine from other professions as well as the boundaries within medicine, and describes the learning of boundaries by medical students.

But how do these erstwhile mortals acquire their infallibility?

> There is a hierarchy. First they are novitiates whose faith is sorely tested by autos-da-fe. They have to burn (in midnight oil) four long years. Thereafter, if not consumed, they enter a monastic order infamous for its asceticism — the "Somnambulists" (in other words, interns). After a year of sleepless penance, they can in turn become flagellators for the younger postulants. And in time, they are initiated. Now there is no limit to their advancement in the Holy Order. Bishop, Cardinal — even the Vatican.
>
> Except in medicine there are ten thousand Romes: the pediatric papacy, the neurological, the psychiatric (whence the term 'spiritual father'). There is even a Sacred Seat for the proctologist. Saint Peter built a church upon a rock. For many doctors, gallstones has sufficed.
>
> But it all commences in ritual humiliation. And be it Buffalo or Boston, Mississippi or Montana, the rites are similar. Those who aspire to face the agony and suffering of humankind must first themselves become acquainted with it (Segal, 1988, p. 84).

Learning Professional Boundaries in Medicine

Learning the boundaries, much like pledge training in a social fraternity, is part of the socialization process of becoming a physician. Both fraterni-

73

ties and medicine have had to yield to external pressures to admit ethnic minorities to their ranks. External pressures have caused social fraternities to eliminate hazing, and public concern for the long hours worked by house staff has caused hospitals to reduce the working hours of students in training. Nonetheless, the boundaries that characterize the elitism of physicians and "actives" in fraternities are inculcated in young neophytes from the beginning. Both social fraternities and medicine are institutions with histories and power bases that are carefully coddled by alumni.

In essence, each discipline in the health field has its own history, training requirements, and boundaries, which make it a specialty. Indeed, it is through the period of training that health professionals learn, not what they have in common with other health professions, but what makes them unique and different. Each discipline creates its own power base and ascribed status, irrespective of whether or not the discipline can function without a physician's supervision. Of course, how powerful or prestigious a profession is, is a matter of the congruence between two sets of perceptions, how one's field is rated by one's peers and how it is seen by non-members.

Jonas (1978) pointed out that most American medical schools tend to be inner directed, setting policies to meet the perceived needs of the schools' faculties and administrators. They have not been proactive in meeting society's changing needs. For example, the schools educating health professionals have maintained a disease-oriented curriculum in the face of society's concern with health and prevention. Most new medical technology is designed to assist in diagnosis and cure; advancements in how to maintain or enhance one's health are left to others outside the scope of medical practice. Much of the public's dissatisfaction with health and medical care is due to premature and inappropriate mobilization of expensive technology on behalf of ordinary problems. This is the result of an educational process that is a synthesis of specialties (Jonas, 1978).

The elaborate rituals and shibboleths evident in the education of physicians, which are described by Jonas and Segal, are luxuries that society cannot afford much longer. Various studies have shown that much of the work of primary care physicians can be performed effectively by other health care professionals (Mauksch, 1978), such as physician's assistants, nurse practitioners, and midwives, whose incomes are generally much lower than those of physicians. It is hard to justify a health care system that provides expensive intensive care units for patients in their last six months of life, but fails to immunize infants against dangerous diseases that are easily preventable. Students and residents are willing to work backbreaking hours and borrow huge amounts of money if the outcomes of these efforts lead to substantial economic gains. However, if economic changes lower the prestige and incomes of physicians, the system will change. Colwill (1992) has indicated that the recruitment of primary care physicians is dropping. Such declines will accelerate unless governmental action is taken. Such actions will alter the entire system.

Allied Health Professionals

The Institute of Medicine (1989) reported that a computerized search of the nation's newspapers for October, 1987, found the term "allied health" in two stories. During the same period, there were 443 references to nursing and more than 500 references to physicians. The scarcity of references reflects a lack of public awareness and of recognition by other health professionals of the more than 200 disciplines that comprise allied health. Despite the continuing debate about definitions and boundaries, some groups of practitioners have come together and unequivocally called themselves allied health personnel. The groups coalesce into three major settings: (1) academic institutions under schools of allied health, to benefit from multidisciplinary interaction and educational efficiency; (2) health service settings, for reasons of personnel administration; and (3) professional associations, to attempt to influence policy, collect information, and publish scholarly papers on issues of interest across the fields. The groups also come together for political reasons. Each profession is small compared to medicine and nursing. Therefore, cooperation gives them more "clout" in terms of resources and bargaining power. Lacking a satisfying definition of allied health, many groups have tried to impose order with a variety of classification schemes. They have been classified, according to departmental affiliation, into such categories as dental, dietary, emergency, diagnostic, and therapeutic.

One study emphasized certain features that cut across different types of work and recommended classification according to patient, laboratory, administration, and community oriented groupings (Bureau of Health Manpower, 1967). A poll of professional organizations arrived at three clusters according to job function: (1) primary care workers; (2) health promotion, rehabilitation, and administration personnel; and (3) test-oriented workers (National Commission on Allied Health Education, 1980). There is no correct taxonomy of allied health. Therefore, in its national study of allied health, the Institute of Medicine emphasized six characteristics of allied health occupations: (1) level of autonomy—some allied health fields have a history of practice without direct physician supervision, others are struggling for independent practice; (2) dependence on technology—those allied health disciplines that are totally dependent upon machines are more vulnerable to job obsolescence than those disciplines that are not so totally dependent; (3) substitutability of personnel—allied health disciplines vary as to how well their turf is marked and protected. If workers from two occupations, or two levels of the same occupation, can perform the same functions, the workers who are paid more, or who are more specialized, may be displaced; (4) flexibility in location of employment—allied health personnel who can work in a variety of settings are less vulnerable in a job market that responds to altered financing incentives by shifting the location of care or by limiting the amount of care provided in some settings; (5) degree of regulation—if a field is highly regulated, employers are constrained from having anyone but workers from that field perform a function. These workers are protected from substitution by other personnel; (6) inclusion in facility accreditation or certification standards—to receive accreditation or certification, a health care facility may be required to employ practitioners in certain fields. If so, the demand for these workers will respond to changes in the number of these facilities.

While the boundaries between allied health personnel and their relationships with physicians, nurses, and other health workers are complex, boundaries within disciplines are based on the required years of preparation. These boundaries establish what allied health practitioners in each discipline can and cannot do. Boundaries within and between allied health disciplines are continually in flux: some groups seek to become more independent from physician supervision; and new fields of specialization, which arose in response to new technologies, threaten to take away tasks that were allocated to other allied health disciplines when diagnosis and treatment were less sophisticated.

The spectrum of allied health, today, includes fields at different stages of evolution. Some allied health fields made the transition from hospital training to baccalaureate education in universities and colleges during the first half of the century. Within the community college movement, in the 1960's, assistant-level programs developed to meet the growing demand for services and the need to make practitioners more productive. The growing demand for services was stimulated by new technology and the availability of funds to pay for new technical services. Medicare, and the increase in life span that was stimulated by more effective treatments for chronic diseases, especially heart disease and hypertension, created a huge demand for physical therapists and occupational therapists. In other fields, the transition to education in academia was made more slowly, for example, radiography and respiratory therapy, which are just now evolving toward requiring a baccalaureate degree. We see some one-year programs giving way to two-year baccalaureate programs and some baccalaureate degree programs evolving toward requiring a Master's degree. As the degree requirements and curriculum content of these fields change, so do the types of jobs graduates will seek. Many individuals with advanced degrees seek administrative jobs, leaving persons with lower levels of training to provide patient care. Boundary realignments will be needed within and between allied health professions to accommodate new graduates with new and expanded skills.

Because of the increasing demands for new skills created by new technology and new knowledge, the number of specialized workers will continue to increase. However, the way they are used may change in order to deal with economic realities. Before the Henry Ford era, most manufacturing was done by skilled workers such as carpenters and machinists. Ford taught each worker a particular task and filled the worker's days with continual repetition of the single task. This enabled him to build cars with less skilled workers. Many health care facilities for indigent patients use only a few physicians who supervise a group of workers with less training, such as nurse practitioners or physician's assistants. Private insurance companies may adopt such a model as health care costs increase, lessening the demand for highly trained professionals. Such a model already exists in mental health facilities, where the shortage of psychiatrists and the cost of their services has encouraged a reliance upon psychologists and psychiatric social workers, under the supervision of psychiatrists, to deliver most of the direct patient care.

Primary care clinics staffed by nurse practitioners, and mental health facilities staffed by clinical psychologists, preserve the traditional hierarchical position of the physician as leader. However, in some settings, there has been a major shift from hierarchy to a system in which physicians share the power for decision-making with other health professionals (Trier, 1985). In team approaches, other health professionals assume a large share of the responsibility for patient care, a share that has increased at the expense of the physician's share (Freddi, 1989). The recent self-awareness and militancy of other health professionals only partially explain the reasons why physicians have lost much of their power. The central condition for change is represented by the organizational and technological complexity of contemporary health care: the physician alone can no longer cope with the scope of new tasks.

Fagin (1992) has documented the many ways that collaboration among nurses and physicians has improved patient care and lowered costs. She reports, however, that attempts to study the effectiveness of nurse/physician collaboration were terminated when the American Medical Association withdrew from a research study of nurse/physician collaboration because of emerging issues regarding expanded roles for nurses and higher salaries commensurate with their professional status. Increasing nurse/physician collaboration will be difficult because it breaks long established boundaries.

Health Personnel Shortages

Ginzberg (1978) has labeled certain beliefs regarding health personnel "sacred cows" because he does not believe they are necessarily true: (1) additional health personnel will result in improved care and health; (2) a serious maldistribution of health personnel exists and is causing hardships; (3) the recruitment of women and members of ethnic minorities will yield significant advantages to the health care system; (4) physicians in private practice underutilize their skills because of insufficient paramedical assistants; and (5) there are too many specialists and too few general practitioners. While we agree with many of Ginsberg's generalizations, we have added some additional comments related to our understanding of the sources of problems with the education and employment of health care workers.

Ginsberg states, and we agree, that health manpower in the U.S. is akin to a rollercoaster gone out of control. We seem to vacillate between shortages and an oversupply. No long-range manpower planning provides for an even flow and even mix of health personnel. The various levels of government pay huge amounts for health care, but, until recently, have shown little interest in controlling costs. The normal constraints of the market do not exist. A similar problem, in the case of savings and loan institutions, led to the massive, expensive collapse of the whole system. The health care system is subject to massive demands for services without any control of costs. A continual demand for more health care workers to staff the system existed for many years without regard to a rational system for distributing health care services. Because of the power and influence of the individual health professions, health care services still focus around the individual skills of practitioners. With some specific exceptions, such as cleft palate and craniofacial teams, there is little or no interdisciplinary care. Health care has become so specialized that a shortage or oversupply of certain types of health professionals can cause a crisis. For example, a shortage of respiratory therapists could put so much strain on a hospital that it might have to limit care or close beds. In instances where two closely related allied health disciplines have similar skills, as in the case of occupational therapy and physical therapy, a shortage in one may be covered by the skills of the other. However, the health care system of accreditation, certification, and licensure discourages the training of individuals in cross-disciplinary activity.

Ginsberg calls the belief that additional health manpower will result in improved care and health idealistic, saying that it is not the number of available health professionals, but how they practice, that influences the quality of care or whether prevention is practiced. Similarly, he calls the serious maldistribution of health manpower a sacred cow, saying that there are never enough health professionals in rural areas and urban ghettos. If health care needs change continually, changing the distribution of health professionals simply represents an attempt to maintain a rough balance between supply and need. No fixed number of health professionals can eliminate the supposed maldistribution problem. The dilemma is one of determining what is needed to meet current needs.

We agree with Ginsberg that increasing the supply of health professionals *by itself* will solve few problems. The supply of health professionals is linked, however, to the economics of health care. If we increase the availability of health care by devising new sources of health care funding, as happened with Medicare and Medicaid, and do nothing about the maldistribution of health workers, the new demands on existing health personnel will cause their salaries to soar. The system of educating health workers has to be understood within the context of health care financing and delivery. If we move to a system that relies on allied health and nursing personnel to be the first contact health providers for millions of people, the salaries of these individuals will increase until the maldistribution of such individuals is solved. Unfortunately, the United States has not been very good at comprehensive planning, even in situations in which government resources are bound to exert a great influence on the entire system.

Ginsberg believes that the recruitment of women and members of ethnic minorities is also a sacred cow. Supposedly, these groups would help remedy shortages and maldistribution problems. But women and members of ethnic minorities want to practice where everyone else does. These groups should be recruited to the health professions because it is right that opportunities be available to all who qualify; however, according to Ginsberg, they will not change the problems of health manpower, significantly.

The government has increased the amount of money available from Medicaid for maternal and child health. These funds have led to the development and improvement of family planning clinics, which are expanding to include postnatal care for women and infants. These clinics are staffed mainly by nurse practitioners and female physicians. Part time practice is very attractive to female physicians, many of whom seek careers that allow them to balance practice with the raising of families. If part-time female physicians were not available, it is likely that these new clinics would not be feasible. This example also illustrates the point that one type of change in itself will not improve the system. Change is required in the system as a whole.

Similarly, the development of more minority health care professionals will not by itself solve work force distribution problems. However, it is unlikely that many non-minority health care workers will be attracted to minority neighborhoods, or that city-bred health workers will be attracted to rural areas. However, *if economic incentives are changed*, the health services available to underserved areas may be bolstered considerably by ethnic minority and rural-bred health workers.

Ginsberg also regards the statement that there are too many specialists and not enough generalists, a sacred cow. He believes, and we agree, that it will be difficult to train enough generalists if they must gain entrance to and survive an educational system that is geared to educating specialists. Generalists must have different goals than specialists and must be satisfied with different rewards. As long as the educational system is in the hands of specialists who pursue their own interests and create their own boundaries, it is unlikely that more generalists will be trained. We believe that the present ways of paying for health care have greatly supported the interests of specialists, since the fee-for-service system of reimbursement strongly supports specialists who can charge a premium for their services.

A Health Maintenance Organization (HMO) system of health care, which charges each patient a flat sum of money despite the services used, discourages the utilization of specialists because they are more costly to the system. Another sacred cow of health manpower utilization, according to Ginsberg, is that physicians underutilize paramedical personnel because there are not enough of them. It is likely that physicians are influenced in their willingness to employ allied health or nurse practitioners by their degree of self-confidence in their own knowledge and skills and their willingness to share decision-making for the benefit of the patient. Expanded roles assign to these practitioners some skills that previously were restricted to physicians, and many physicians do not feel secure in acknowledging that allied health or nurse practitioners can perform some skills better than they can (Freidson, 1975). The authors have observed that the best endorsement for a physician's assistant or nurse practitioner comes from the doctor who has experienced the benefits of employing one. While Ginsberg's analysis is accurate, it is based on the assumption that the health care system will continue in its present pattern. Physicians hire physician extenders not only based on their perceived competencies, but also on the perceived economic gains. The physician must be able to bill for the extender's services in ways that increase the physician's economic status. As the number of physicians increases, and the ability of patients to pay decreases, physicians' willingness to hire extenders decreases. For example, one of the authors recently learned that his dentist had decided, when his dental hygienist left his employment, not to hire a new one. Since he paid the hygienist a salary, he had to keep her busy all the time. The hygienist's appointments failed to keep up with her salary, and the dentist's workday was not crowded, so he opted to do some of the cleaning himself and refer other patients to a periodontist.

The supply of physician extenders will increase when they are used to replace physicians, not to help them. Such replacement is already occurring in large indigent care facilities and clinics for Medicaid patients. If second tier systems for health services continue to expand along with Medicaid, or in response to a government mandated second tier system for medically indigent patients, demands for paramedical personnel will increase and the market for physician services will decrease.

Health personnel shortages create new anxieties about turf among the members of a discipline that cannot educate enough professionals fast enough, especially if the discipline, itself, is expanding its boundaries. For example, physical therapy is encouraging its members, especially faculty members, to obtain doctoral degrees and engage in research. These are new roles for physical therapists, and create new opportunities for physical therapy to interface with other disciplines as well as to expand its own knowledge base. Yet, these changes create the need for physical therapists to realign their boundaries with those of related practitioners, such as occupational therapists, health and fitness specialists, orthopedists, and psychiatrists. Meanwhile, there is an acute shortage of practicing physical therapists to provide patient care. Classes of students engaged in Master's level work must be limited because of the limited number of faculty members who are qualified to supervise Master's degree students. Therefore, the supply of new graduates from existing physical therapy programs cannot meet the current demand for therapists.

Physical therapy provides an interesting example of how following medicine's model and using educational limitations to control the training of future practitioners can benefit those already in practice by limiting the supply of new practitioners. This model assures well trained graduates and helps facilitate research and development in the areas of competence controlled by the practitioners. On the other hand, the shortage of physical therapists and the high cost of their services might deny indigent patients any such benefits and severely restrict the benefits available to patients, such as those with Medicaid, who have inadequate insurance. This may, in turn, result in an expansion of the number of physical therapy aides and other second tier workers, who are not licensed physical therapists, but perform some rehabilitative services. A similar phenomenon has occurred in the mental health field. A number of therapists have emerged. Many of them, such as clinical psychologists and psychiatric social workers, are licensed. Others, who do not claim to be therapists, also address mental health problems.

The Cost of Health Care

Health care takes a large portion of our Gross National Product, a larger portion than that of any other country. Paradoxically, we leave a large portion of our population without an identified insurer or with inadequate insurance provided by Medicaid, the Federal government's program of partnership with the States for providing health care for the poor. The reasons for this anomoly lie in how our health care system is financed and the boundaries that have emerged to protect the special interests that have evolved. These special interests include: the elderly, who have a government sponsored health care system; insurance companies, which receive a percentage of health care costs; health care workers, especially physicians, who have seen their incomes soar since third party payment systems become dominant in American health care; unionized workers, government workers, and employees of large businesses, which have systems that are partly financed by employers; and health science centers, which have large numbers of private patients. Losers in this system are the poor, whose health care is controlled by state and local governments; the state and local governments, whose costs have soared; individuals who work for small businesses; and the self-employed. While many employers welcomed the system, initially, since it allowed them to increase wages by paying employees with non-tax dollars, disillusionment set in when costs began to soar.

Health care is expensive for many reasons: its high-tech nature, the cost of specialists, the localization of expertise and equipment in urban areas, the focus on diagnosis and treatment, and the large number of clients with chronic diseases, many associated with aging and lifestyle, for which there is no cure. It is also expensive because incentives to control costs are very weak in fee-for-service systems of reimbursement. Physicians have incentives to overtreat and to order expensive tests and procedures. The high cost of care means that it is available, accessible, and affordable only to persons who have some form of health insurance. Forty million Americans do not have health insurance. Therefore, a clear boundary separates those who seek and receive health care from those who delay or deny their health care needs. There is also a clear boundary between users of health care services and users of Health Maintenance Organizations. The latter are usually more concerned about maintaining and enhancing their state of health. Boundaries separate health professionals who work for Health Maintenance Organizations from health professionals who are in solo or other group practice arrangements. There are also natural boundaries between generalists and specialists with respect to the cost of health care, and there are boundaries between health professionals who can be reimbursed by Medicare and those who cannot.

Perhaps the greatest boundary, with respect to the cost of health care, is that between the amount of dollars we are willing to spend for health versus the amount we wish to spend on other priorities (Fuchs, 1986). The basic question is not what kind of health care system can we afford, but what kind of health care system do we want? Cost will be controlled once the societal goal is established, in contrast to the current situation, in which the cost boundaries of health care keep expanding, gradually eliminating increasing numbers of Americans from crossing the boundary of cost (Fein, 1986). Unfortunately, average Americans and average voters have difficulty answering a question about what kind of health care system they want. Various special interests have helped develop the present system, and those interests continue to exercise power and authority. Americans tend to favor incremental approaches to solving public policy issues, but incremental solutions to the problems of health care access, tend to increase health care costs.

Boundary Conflicts

Conflict is incompatible behavior between parties whose interests differ (Brown, 1983). Conflict may be either good or bad, depending on the circumstances and the values of the observer. Conflict management can require intervention to reduce conflict, if there is too much, or intervention to promote conflict, if there is too little. Most managers regard conflict as a problem to be defused or suppressed as quickly as possible. However, some conflict is necessary in organizations to inspire a search for alternatives and mobilize resources and energies. Conflict often occurs at organizational interfaces, at the link between parties. As organizations become more specialized and larger, there are more interfaces and more opportunities for conflict to occur.

As the inevitable cost squeeze relating to health care emerges, conflict among higher and lower cost professionals is bound to increase. Health Maintenance Organizations prefer family physicians to specialists and, in the future, may depend more and more on physician extenders. While reliance on lesser trained professionals may lower costs and facilitate access to health care, it may also inhibit incentives for higher levels of educational accomplishment and for research and development in the field of health care.

Conflicts Within Professional Groups

Hankin (1989) describes how general dentists, who refer patients to specialists in good economic times, are less likely to refer in a tight economy. New or newly popularized procedures, such as the current one involving implants, often lead to turf wars. Many individuals believe that implants should be limited to oral surgeons and periodontists, but, in actuality, thousands of general practitioners are involved in implant dentistry, to the point of having organized a new dental specialty called "implantology."

Serrett (1985) discusses the several boundary shifts that have occurred throughout the history of occupational therapy and the current division in the profession between practitioners, who are searching for more on the job skills, and the profession's leaders, who are encouraging members to develop theories and conduct research. According to Serrett, "One way to reconcile these opposing forces is to develop a principle that both groups can deeply commit to and support" (p. 27). Other forces outside occupational therapy are also creating a shift in tasks for the entire profession. Serrett states,

> ...A sea (of) change is occurring in our environments, one that has to do...
> with accountability for results. We are currently witnessing the transformation
> of health and human services into businesses ... The managerial demands on
> occupational therapists in mental health have accelerated. Most therapists are
> both delivering direct services to clients and carrying out increasing responsi-
> bilities for managerial tasks ... promotional opportunities are opening for
> those who do well in the managerial areas and those who can facilitate efficient
> and effective team accomplishment. Thus, there is real opportunity in these
> shifting times (p. 3).

Sometimes the strongest threat to turf comes from within. Preparation for professional practice in nursing is largely in non-baccalaureate programs. The American Nurse's Association supports two levels of nursing: professional and technical. It recommends that those wishing to practice professional nursing obtain a bachelor's degree and be called registered nurses, and those who wish to practice technical nursing obtain an associate degree and be called associate nurses. Nurses who already have a license to practice as registered nurses would be grandfathered into the professional category. Nursing has tried to eliminate the Licensed Practical Nurse (LPN) level of nursing because the LPN schools are dominated by hospitals. Recently, the American Medical Association tried to develop a new nursing category called Registered

Care Technician (RCT), a position which resembled that of the LPN, because of an acute shortage of bedside nurses. Such shortages were especially acute in nursing homes, which could not afford to hire even technical nurses and relied heavily on LPN's. The AMA hoped the RCT would attract males to nursing careers and also offer opportunities to low income aspirants to nursing careers who could not afford to attend junior colleges. The conflict between the AMA and the nursing profession over the RCT seemed to abate when the nursing profession agreed to allow the LPN occupation to continue (American Medical Association, 1989).

Westra (1986) points out turf threats from outside nursing. Doctors might try to "recapture" certain nursing responsibilities, such as physical assessments, which were once considered medicine's turf. Proposed changes in some nurse practice acts suggest that this retrenchment has begun. Nurse-midwives and practitioners, for example, are fighting legislation that would require them to practice under a doctor's supervision and, in some states, under regulations set by medical practice boards.

But, as Westra (1986) continues, "holding our own in professional turf battles doesn't simply entail defending what we have now. As the health scene changes, we must search for ways to expand our turf in the right direction. . . . We must continually ask ourselves, "Why shouldn't we take on this task?" (p. 53).

Conflicts Between Professional Groups

Dentistry and Dental Auxiliaries. Morganstein (1989) details the historical development of dental auxiliaries and the "turf" associated with various dental groups. He notes that the establishment of dentistry as a profession was a battle for turf. In England, in the early 1500's, most dental surgery was performed by barbers; most physicians considered extracting teeth below their dignity. Rivalry between surgeons and barbers was intense until the two groups met and agreed they could not perform each other's skills. Dentistry, in America, in the 1600's and 1700's, was practiced by "tooth drawers," barbers, and blacksmiths. In the early 1800's, the best surgeon-dentists began to limit their trade to dentistry alone. Maryland became the first state to regulate the practice of dentistry when, in 1805, regulatory authority for physicians was expanded to include dentists. By the mid-1800's, some dentists were receiving a portion of their training in medical schools. In 1840, dentists established the first dental college in the world in Baltimore after failing to convince the medical school faculty to increase the curriculum time for the dental program.

Dentistry flourished. In the late 1800's, dentists began to use chair-side dental assistants. The role of the assistant gradually expanded to include receptionist duties and the performance of laboratory procedures. In the early 1900's, two types of dental auxiliaries evolved: the dental hygienist who assisted the dentist in cleaning teeth, and the dental laboratory technician who performed procedures that included making false teeth. All states licensed dentists by 1935 and began to license hygienists during the 1920's. Dental assistants and dental laboratory technicians are not licensed. The dental assistant performs chair-side assistance and related office and laboratory procedures under the direction and supervision of a dentist. Although dental assistants are not required to complete formal training programs, such programs are available and have been accredited nationally since 1960.

Dental hygienists serve as oral health technicians and educators to help the public develop and maintain optimal oral health. The dental hygienist performs preventive and therapeutic patient care under the supervision of the dentist. In contrast to dental assistants, dental hygienists are required to complete an accredited educational program for licensure. Dental hygiene programs have been accredited nationally since 1952.

The dental lab technician performs laboratory procedures in the manufacture of prosthetic appliances under the written authorization of the dentist. Accreditation standards for training dental laboratory technicians were developed in 1946.

In 1963, the Health Professions Education Assistance Act was passed with the primary intent of providing funds to construct new health professions schools and expand existing ones. The number of dental schools in the United States expanded from 47, in 1962, to 60, in 1979. The Allied Health Professions Personnel Training Act, passed in 1966, created an increase from 58 to 179 dental hygiene training programs and from 81 to 262 dental assisting programs between 1966 and 1976.

During the 1960's and 1970's, while the numbers of dentists and auxiliaries were expanding, numerous studies were conducted concerning the use of dental assistants and dental hygienists in an expanded capacity. Studies consistently demonstrated that productivity increased 80–140% when dental auxiliary personnel were used. Dental auxiliaries were pleased, while dentists were not. The American Dental Association, which had originally supported studies concerning the expanded use of dental auxiliaries, changed its practice acts to restrict the expanded functions of some dental auxiliaries. By 1980, almost all states had made such changes. The number of dentists and dental auxiliaries were exploding. The national economy was declining and dental business was at its lowest point in years. The American Dental Association initiated policies encouraging greater restrictions in the expanded functions of auxiliaries. While the auxiliary functions were stabilized, territoriality within the dental profession began to emerge between various sections of the dental assistant group, between dental laboratory technicians and dentists, and between dental hygienists and dentists.

The challenge for turf first came from laboratory technicians in Canada when a number of laboratory technicians, authorized to make dental impressions under the supervision of a dentist, began to perform these functions on their own. These individuals became known as "denturists." In the mid 1970's, this movement spread to the United States. Between 1980 and 1985, Oregon, Idaho, and Montana, through voter initiative followed by legislative endorsement, approved laws permitting the performance of these procedures by laboratory technicians with no supervisory restrictions after two years of training and a two-year internship.

A controversy was initiated by dental hygienists in California, in 1976, when one hygienist opened an office adjacent to that of her former employer, a dentist. In that case, Attorney General vs. Linda Krol, Krol was considered an independent contractor delivering services to patients of contracting dentists and, therefore, under the "general supervision" of dentists. In 1985, the American Dental Association's Council on Dental Education initiated a review of policies on dental auxiliaries, which has led to more specificity and greater control by dentists.

Since 1975, the number of applicants to dental schools has declined substantially as has the number of applications to dental auxiliary programs. Now, dentistry faces a crisis. Dental schools and programs for auxiliaries find it difficult to fill their classes. At the same time, there is a shortage of dental auxiliaries. Dentists and dental laboratories are finding it difficult to hire well qualified assistants, hygienists, and technicians. In response, the American Dental Association has implemented a project to attract a pool of highly qualified candidates to dental and dental auxiliary programs to ensure an adequate supply of dental personnel to meet the further needs of the population. The lessons learned from dentistry suggest that technicians' roles, in regard to functions, training, recognition, legal status, and supervision, should be clearly defined, and the professions intimately involved in establishing them.

Medicine and Pharmacy. In both England and the United States, physicians and pharmacists carry out functionally related tasks, but observe a boundary of power and task division that is legally and ethically enforced. Furthermore, the pharmacists' code of ethics enjoins them from encroaching on physicians' task territory: they should not prescribe drugs nor diagnose illness. Although physicians are legally and ethically prevented from collecting payment for drugs, they can still dispense them, and they give away free samples from drug manufacturers. A few states prohibit physicians from owning pharmacies and benefitting financially from prescribing.

In the American colonies, in the early 1700's, physicians actually were informally trained apothecary-surgeons who ran dispensaries to help support themselves since their clients were too poor for practitioners to survive solely on fees (Kronus, 1976). The Revolutionary War provided the economic impetus for the first separation of apothecary from medical roles. Toward the end of the 18th Century, state regulations favoring the monopoly of formally educated doctors were passed. Rather than prohibiting apothecaries, surgeons, and druggists from prescribing drugs, these regulations set standards for apprenticeships and examinations.

Medical societies made several early attempts to regulate the practice of druggists and other untrained medical practitioners. Beleaguered druggists responded, in many cases, by forming protective associations to combat threatening legislation or invalidate the physicians' right to claim control in the absence of an occupational organization (Kronus, 1976). In fact, the first pharmacy association was formed to combat the physicians' attempts to assume regulatory power over druggists. The code of ethics adopted by the American Pharmaceutical Association in 1862 simply recommended a separation of functions: "the members of this Association. . . . in conducting business at the counter, should avoid prescribing for disease when applicable, referring applicants for medical advice to the physician." Stronger language was used to prevent boundary crossing by physicians:

> We also consider that the practice of some physicians . . . of obtaining medicines at low prices . . . and selling them to their patients, is not only unjust and unprofessional, but deserving the censure of all high-minded medical men (Kronus, 1976).

In the 1912 version of the American Medical Association's Code of Ethics, only two sentences were devoted to relationships with pharmacists. The difference in these ethical codes clearly indicates the disparity in power. Although boundaries, in practice, were and still are traversed informally by pharmacists, physicians controlled pharmacists' resources in knowledge and training.

The post-war "drug explosion," and the thalidomide tragedy, generally expanded public awareness of the problems of iatrogenesis and drug use. Certain pharmacists claimed that, with a knowledge of the pharmaceutical sciences, they could help to promote a safer, more effective use of drugs. Attempts to expand pharmacy's role to encompass the clinical dimension are not new. Clinical pharmacy and clinical pharmacology groups within pharmacy and medicine are committed to changing certain aspects of the system of drug use. Pharmacy is encompassing more clinical subjects in its curriculum and offering physicians expanded services in advising the selection of prescribed drugs. Clinical pharmacologists are not a threat to medicine. Clinical experience and the notion that diagnosis and treatment cannot be separated remain the defensive ideology of the medical profession. (Uzych, 1988).

Although specialism may appear to produce strains and tensions within a professional body, these are contained and stabilized, and do not threaten the autonomy of the profession as a whole. Specialism is a way of ordering and controlling semiautonomous segments, structured so that ties and allegiances do not conflict (Eaton and Webb, 1979). Having acknowledged such problems in drug use as iatrogenesis, noncompliance, and adverse drug effects, the medical profession has defined those problems so as to allow only a medical solution. The emergence of clinical pharmacology as a specialty has enabled the medical profession to defend its autonomy by claiming to have set its own house in order (Eaton and Webb, 1979).

A significant number of issues, in which the practicing pharmacist's judgment has an immediate effect that goes beyond competence, legality, or the general norms in ethical codes, will grow in importance in the future. For example, pressure to allow the pharmacist to use drugs that are the bioequivalent of those prescribed is now increasing, as is a movement toward generic prescribing in which the pharmacist may exercise a choice. Codes related to addictive drugs have placed upon pharmacists, when it comes to their attention, the responsibility for preventing incipient addiction. This gives pharmacists additional moral responsibility and opens up the possibility of conflict with patients and physicians. Products sold over the counter also present pharmacists with ethical choices. In the future, especially if new classes of drugs that can be sold by pharmacists are developed, the ethical problems inherent in prescribing will be experienced increasingly by pharmacists. Like their present responsibilities regarding the dispensing of narcotic drugs, pharmacists will assume special obligations when dispensing mind-altering drugs, drugs that can easily be abused. The pharmacist cannot refuse a prescription without coming face to face with a physician who may resent the pharmacist's counsel and without being prepared to face irate patients who see their privacy being invaded (Reich, 1978, pp. 1211–1214).

The role of pharmaceutical services in our health care system is evolving. The traditional functions of the pharmacist have been altered markedly.

Occupational Therapy and Physical Medicine. Occupational therapy and physical medicine have had a tenuous relationship since physical medicine was organized following World War II. As physiatrists organized and sought specialty status, they directly challenged occupational therapy's autonomy within the health care system. At its 1946 annual meeting, the Occupational Therapy Board discussed a document from the U.S. Public Health Service that required occupational and physical therapy to function under one department in U.S. Marine hospitals. The document seemingly highlighted an effort to fit occupational therapy into a physical medicine mold (Colman, 1992). Additional evidence was provided by the fact that physiatrists were being trained in techniques considered occupational therapy.

During the 1946 to 1947 academic year, several members of a committee of physiatrists approached the University of Illinois Medical School in Chicago about developing a physical medicine division. The head of occupational therapy was involved in the discussions, in which the physiatrists proposed a relationship similar to that they enjoyed with physical therapy: the control of their education and their registry of therapists. The physiatrists offered the occupational therapy department a grant to support a clinical director. This plan was rejected; nonetheless, the physiatrists attempted to gain control of occupational therapy at the University of Illinois through petitions to the administration and pressure for restructuring that placed occupational therapy under physical medicine's jurisdiction (Colman, 1992).

The struggle of occupational therapy to retain its autonomy has continued. In the 1950's, the physiatrists, while agreeing that medical supervision of occupational therapy students need not be conducted by a physiatrist, continued to object to the term, *therapist,* claiming that it implied diagnosis, and suggested that the label, occupational therapy *technician,* be substituted for occupational therapist.

Occupational therapy has made at least two compromises in its relationship with physiatrists. The discipline's essentials now state that occupational therapy schools can be sited at medical schools and that the clinical training portion of the entry-level education program in occupational therapy can be directed by an individual or a committee of physicians (Colman, 1992).

Occupational therapy's struggle for survival took on new dimensions in the 1990's. Five of the oldest programs in the United States, all part of major research universities, recently closed or were put under consideration for closure. Survival in an academic environment involves the need for research, doctoral level faculty, and programs that meet the criteria for an academic discipline and contribute to the universe of knowledge. Occupational therapy programs do not conform to the rules of an academic environment and are, therefore, being threatened (Yerxa, 1991). Occupational therapy, within its boundaries, has not developed a model of an integrated discipline. Practice is viewed as its totality. As Yerxa (1991) has said, "what we have rather than an integrated discipline is practice and education linked in a closed loop, that is a short circuit robbing occupational therapy of the power needed to do our best for patients."

To become an integrated discipline, occupational therapy needs to develop a knowledge base. At present, occupational therapy derives its knowledge from numerous other disciplines, e.g., art and recreational therapy, ergonomics, psychology, psychiatry, orthotics, and others. To become an integrated discipline, occupational therapy will need to develop core theories and conduct the necessary research to test these theories. Currently, occupational therapy does not have the research infrastructure or clinician-researchers to move ahead quickly with the development of a knowledge base.

Once the knowledge base of occupational therapy has been defined, its relationship with other, closely related disciplines will become clearer. Occupational therapists who conduct activities that overlap those of other disciplines, such as social work, nursing, or orthopedics, run the risk of not being taken seriously because they lack credentials in a particular area. One way occupational therapists have coped with bound-ary problems in their discipline is by specializing or subspecializing, thereby limiting their contact with a variety of disciplines and working with a small cadre of professionals who know their abilities and skills in the clinical arena.

Almost all of the major issues facing occupational therapy over the next decade involve boundaries—the manpower shortage, educational changes, ethical and legal issues, payment for services, credibility, and the philosophy of the profession (Bruhn, 1991). Boundaries are often thought of as barriers, but they can be opportunities. Boundary issues within occupational therapy involve therapists and assistants, practi-tioners and educators, traditionalists and opportunists. Boundary issues with occupational therapy involve some 19 other professions including physical therapy, nursing, social work, and art and music therapy. Occu-pational therapy is, therefore, probably more subject to economic pres-sures than physical therapy, which has less competition for the type of services it delivers.

Physical Therapy and Medicine. Like other health occupations in the United States, physical therapy is undergoing expansion and striving for professional status. Role expansion is occurring horizontally; there are increases in the types of practice sites and the number of procedures administered. Role expansion is also occurring vertically; many new or modified procedures require greater degrees of practitioner compe-tency, and autonomous decisions (Ritchey *et al.*, 1989). Since autonomy is the decisive dimension of professional status enhancement, and since the physician has traditionally held the dominant role in medical care, vertical role expansion by other health professions must adapt to the structure of physician practice. Physician control over physical therapy is evident in the state laws governing physical therapy practice. Ritchey *et al.*, (1989) report that the functional aspect of physicians' knowledge is the decisive variable in increasing referrals to physical therapists, and that an emphasis on status issues by physical therapy associates, at this time, may be counterproductive. Vertical role expansion of physical therapy is likely to occur quietly in the workplace and in contract negotiations with insurance companies rather than in the statehouse (Ritchey *et al.*, 1989). While physicians and physical therapists are not waging a turf battle, there is competition for task jurisdiction. As new technologies and techniques arise, the medical profession will regulate them until it is clear the tasks can be delegated. The medical profession is still in a position to strongly influence the professional boundaries of physical therapy, but less able to dictate those boundaries.

The Need for Collaboration

Most of the problems encountered by health care professionals—human abuse, substance abuse, AIDS, the elderly, and the homeless—cannot be handled within the scope of a single discipline. The health problems of the future will grow increasingly complex and the problem-solving, technical, and educational skills of many disciplines will be required to carry out the process of diagnosis, treatment, and rehabilitation. The family and extended family, in its many forms, rather than one identified client, increasingly will be the focus for intervention. Increasingly, health professionals will see that the majority of problems can only be patched up, and that the best intervention is prevention.

Social change that challenges boundaries or territories is basically good; however, the changes that accompany economic stringency can be damaging to the development of new approaches to health care delivery. Whether a profession perceives boundary issues as threats or opportunities depends a lot on how well they have minded their profession. Professions that are perceived to be diffuse and unstable are more likely to be the target of takeovers than professions which have a strong identity and whose members, and persons outside the profession, know the limits of their expertise.

Professions establish boundaries to protect their turf and, therefore, their philosophy, skills, and the things that make them unique. Uniqueness is what helps keep them needed and, as the need exists, they continue to exist. Professions do not need to be adversarial or defensive in order to retain their uniqueness. It is our view that collaboration offers the opportunity to market a profession's uniqueness by letting others know and see what it does well.

The boundary relationship between occupational therapy and physical therapy is used to illustrate some of these points (Figure 3-1). The major theme that occupational therapy and physical therapy share is human movement. Occupational therapy focuses on the social and psychological, cognitive and perceptual aspects of movement, and physical therapy on the physical aspects. Each discipline has skills and areas of focus that distinguish it from the other. Physical therapy's expertise lies in cardiac rehabilitation, gross body ambulation, and sports medicine. Occupa-

FIGURE 3-1

**The Shared and Separate Boundaries
of Occupational Therapy and Physical Therapy**

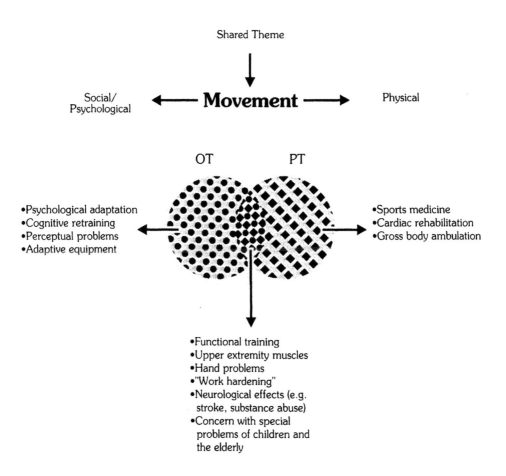

Source: John G. Bruhn

tional therapy's expertise lies in cognitive retraining, perceptual problems, adaptive equipment, and social and psychological aspects of rehabilitation, behavior modification, stress, coping, and energy conservation. The future promises new and exciting opportunities for occupational therapists in discharge planning and sports psychology in collaboration with social workers and physical therapists, respectively. Some health problems, such as neonatal, hand, and burn problems, functional training, and work hardening, require the unique perspectives and skills of both occupational and physical therapists. However, depending on the availability of personnel and the philosophy of the work environment, these issues may generate conflict rather than collaboration.

Conflicts in Defining New Areas of Knowledge

The use of the term, gerontology, has preceded any consensus about its meaning and about the scope and boundaries of a science of aging. In fact, the meanings of gerontology have been in flux for more than a century (Achenbaum and Levin, 1989). A technical term lacking specificity, gerontology has generated controversy about which of its aspects should be emphasized. Aging has been described as a process. Synthesizing motifs hold gerontology to be an integrated understanding of developmental processes over time; however, they have not helped to refine or define critical issues in aging.

The National Institute of Aging has stated that gerontology is the study of aging from the broadest perspective. With such a perspective, virtually no discipline can be excluded from its study. The number of elderly in the United States is growing, making the study of aging politically popular, and funds for research into its many facets are available. While the interdisciplinary nature of gerontology is accepted and lauded, few teaching and research models use the interdisciplinary approach.

Difficulty arises from the fact that gerontology and pediatrics challenge the machine metaphor that has enthralled medicine since the explosive growth of modern science in the last century and a half. This metaphor sees the human body as a machine that can be fixed by medical intervention. Such a view neglects the environment in which the patient lives and the effects of attitudes and self-awareness on the patient. The prognosis for the very old and very young is influenced greatly both by their immediate families and by the communities in which they live. Old people in caring environments, with some simple adjustments of their physical and emotional surroundings, can often make surprisingly effective adjustments to physical and mental disabilities that would "warehouse" their contemporaries in nursing homes. The creation of such environments makes crossdisciplinary demands on health professionals and representatives of the community (Lesnoff-Caraviglia, 1980).

Perhaps it is best that this topic of personal and political interest be studied by many discrete groups, with each group contributing to the general knowledge about aging from it's own particular field of interest. The enormous cost of long term care and the rapid growth of the number of very old people makes this topic one of pressing concern, which will challenge the creativity of the groups involved. Similarly, the problems of developing an appropriate environment for children and adolescents create similar demands for cross-disciplinary discussion, planning and experimentation.

Health professionals draw boundaries when they intervene to respond to illness in geriatric patients. In a study of physicians' roles and boundaries in treating geriatric patients, it was found that physicians were able to provide linkages between acute care treatment and necessary long-term care services through their interactions with their patients (Kaufman and Becker, 1991). Physicians attempted to bridge gaps between medical and emotional needs and clinical and social services with social, psychotherapeutic, and biomedical interventions. These researchers found physicians' activities with stroke patients to be so broadly construed that treatment and management of stroke may be seen as paradigmatic for the role of physicians in long-term care.

An examination of how physicians draw the boundaries of medicine in their roles as primary care providers to elderly patients illustrates the complexity of policy issues in long-term care of the elderly. An active role in long-term care by physicians is sometimes referred to by critics as medicalization. As the definition of geriatric medicine attests, physicians who have elderly patients must look outside the biomedical model to fulfill their treatment goals. Rather than usurp their patients' control or view their problems and needs as diseases, Kaufman and Becker (1991) found that primary care physicians work both as biomedical doctors and as providers of social and emotional support. The perceptions of physicians about the extended boundaries of the primary care role suggest that they view this responsibility as one that is as important as medical treatment.

Boettcher (1985) found that health professionals imposed boundaries of time and space on their patients, especially those in hospitals or nursing homes. Boundary marking was implemented by nursing interventions, medical interventions, institutional policies, Medicare and

Medicaid policies, physical design, and human relationships. The lack of free access to personal space and the establishment of schedules were boundary markers imposed on patients by staff. Boettcher's concern was that a health care environment that proposes to give personal care should be an environment in which the health personnel do their best to fulfill patient needs. Rigid boundaries, imposed knowingly or unknowingly by staff, inhibit patients from expressing their needs.

Clarifying the Boundaries of Practice

The shift in emphasis and reimbursement from acute institutional care to the provision of care in the home has made home nursing care into a growing, constantly changing field of practice. More nurses work in home care today than at any earlier time, yet people are confused about exactly what home nursing care is and how it differs from other home services (Humphrey, 1988).

Nurses and consumers have difficulty understanding the role of community health nurses, particularly since various specialties, such as that of the nurse practitioner, have emerged within the nursing profession. Nursing has set boundaries for professional practice, identifying most of its specialist groups with medical specialties, for example, psychiatric nursing, obstetric nursing, medical-surgical nursing, oncology nursing. Some specialties in nursing, such as geriatric nursing and intensive care nursing, have been defined by population groups and settings. The patients seen by community health and home care nurses are affected by a variety of disease conditions, needs, and environmental factors. Nurses in these practice settings view themselves as generalists. Because of the predominance of specialty practice in nursing, questions often have been raised about the validity of their area of nursing. Community health nursing, because it is a field of generalists, has been involved in boundary conflicts with other nursing specialties.

Practice is only partially defined by the setting in which it takes place (Pritchard, 1989). Internal boundaries, which involve one's self-identity and self-concept, also help define the importance of the work one does. This is especially true for home care nurses since they are not the sole providers of home care. A variety of technical and professional services are provided to patients in the home. The home care professional team is made up of doctors, dentists, nurses, homemakers, home health aides, and physical, speech, occupational, and respiratory therapists, as well as clinical dietitians. High technology health care equipment, including renal dialysis machines, equipment for intravenous infusion therapies, respirators, and other devices, are available for home use. Many specialists have expanded their practice settings to the community and the patient's home, territory that formerly was almost the sole prerogative of the visiting nurse or home health aide. The arrival of diagnostic related groups (DRG's) helped to rearrange, dramatically, the practice boundaries of generalists and specialists (Humphrey, 1988).

Social work, a profession that, traditionally, has had broad boundaries that span the family and its relationships with the social and physical environments in which it exists, is faced with even broader and more complex issues (Abramson and Black, 1985). Life-support systems, organ transplants, and other advances in medical technology have made it possible to prolong life. Recent breakthroughs in treating the fetus also extend the definition of personhood at the beginning of life. As more options and opportunities become available to the patient, a broad framework to guide decision-making becomes a greater necessity to the health professional. Bioethics is now an area of concern for the social work profession. Unlike health professionals, whose patient responsibilities are limited by their practice settings, social workers' responsibilities cover many settings and follow patients and their families over time. It is becoming more difficult to determine when it is time to end a relationship with a client.

Boundary Problems of Generalists

Generalists work in open systems. The boundaries of their practices extend far beyond the physical settings of their practices. Generalists must deal with poorly defined boundaries; therefore, they must be unique individuals who are willing to cope with ambiguity and change. Often, generalists must be proactive rather than reactive; they must be negotiators and managers and have a good self-concept. Generalists, who build networks between people and organizations, work in a climate of cooperation to achieve a client's goal. Therefore, specialists often view generalists as "boundaryless," implying that they lack in-depth knowledge about most topics. Health professionals become specialists intentionally, to limit their boundaries and scope of responsibility. They want more control over their world. Limiting one's boundaries limits one's view of the world. The world views of both the generalist and the specialist are appropriate; however, individuals must avoid being so specialized that they cannot see the relationships among various factors of the patient's world, or so broad that they cannot focus on issues. These extremes make problem solving difficult. One can be an "inter-disciplinarian" and still be a specialist; it's a matter of perspective and self-assurance regarding whom one is and what one knows and does not know.

Patients and Professional Boundaries

Boundaries define the point at which "vulnerability" ends and "at risk" begins (Rose and Killien, 1983; Scott, 1988). Gitterman (1989) discusses how and why patients test authority, assay boundaries, and explore limits in professional relationships. Patients test boundaries through such behaviors as provocation, interruption, seduction, overt hostility, withdrawal, silence, cancellation of appointments, precipitous termination, leaving treatment against medical advice, changing the subject, minimizing issues, withholding information, or denial. The testing of authority, power, and boundaries depends a lot on the *way* in which a patient comes to the health professional. It is likely that the patient who *seeks* help and the professional will be able to mediate and accommodate to mutual expectations. When a physician refers a patient, the authority associated with the referring physician and any ambiguity about the referral often stimulate the patient to engage in behaviors that test the new relationship. Parents may bring a child to a professional for help, but the professional cannot assume that the child wants help. Patients or clients in particular situations may be *mandated* to accept professional help, e.g., probation, adoption. People who are offered or compelled to accept services may test the professional's purposes and creditability.

Patients or clients often test a professional's limits of authority and power. The patient may test to see which side the professional is on before deciding to trust the professional. The patient often seeks the professional's approval and may be sensitive to subtle expressions of approval or disapproval. For example, a patient may be sensitive about aspects of his/her lifestyle or health habits that he/she may not wish to change. Some patients or clients test boundaries to gain personal control. They may want to control their interaction with the professional, tell only what they want to tell, and pressure the professional to give them the type of help or treatment they expect. Differences in social class, ethnicity, race, sex, or stage of development may also stimulate testing behavior. Some patients seek advice and direction; others seek insight and reassurance. Some patients expect immediate solutions to their problems, while others are more tolerant regarding the length of treatment. One reason for testing boundaries is the helping relationship, itself. In many relationships, the patient or client may reenact parental and sibling experiences and transfer thoughts and feelings to the professional. Patients and clients may create excessive demands and create an excessive dependence on the helper (Gitterman, 1989).

Health professionals almost automatically assume the principle of beneficence. This duty to promote good sometimes conflicts with personal and professional boundaries. One expects persons who are ill to comply with treatment to get well, especially if the ill person sought out help. Clients who do not follow the therapist's treatment instructions are labeled noncompliant. Health professionals consider noncompliant patients or clients "bad" because they transgress boundaries and prevent the health professionals from being beneficent. Patients may be noncompliant because misunderstandings exist between them and their helpers—they may not understand the proposed treatment, they may be afraid, they may not have the money, and so on—all issues that the health professionals may not have identified or clarified.

Haddad (1989) discusses another boundary problem that arises after a helping relationship has been established: when to end the relationship and deal with the patient's concerns about being abandoned, especially during home care. Professional standards require that home care providers persevere, even in the face of considerable inconvenience. Home care providers must weigh the duty of fidelity against the risks and hardships involved before terminating a case. When they reach a decision to conclude care, home care providers are ethically obligated to help patients find other providers or an alternative method of care. Problems of abandonment, non-compliance, and futility will increase as the number of chronically ill persons increases. Finding ethical resolutions to these boundary issues is confounded by regulatory and fiscal matters.

Stone (1976) discusses boundary violations between therapist and patient. He focuses particularly on sexual encounters between male psychiatrists and their female patients. When a serious boundary violation between patient and therapist occurs, the subsequent treatment is jeopardized and sometimes ruined. The patient has to interrupt treatment to look for a new therapist, seriously compromising the patient's capacity to trust. Stone (1976) says there can be no substitute for an enlightened public and proposes professional ostracism, including the refusal to refer patients, of colleagues who have breached professional ethics.

Defining the boundaries of professional competence in the health professions is difficult because competence is best viewed on a continuum from highly competent to clearly incompetent. Norman (1985) proposed a schema of clinical competence, describing five domains of professional activities deemed essential to clinical performance: knowledge and understanding, clinical skills, technical skills, problem solving and clinical judgment, and personal attributes. Overholser and Fine (1990) discussed several strategies to prevent professional incompetence. Competence, however, must be seen in the context of the health care setting. New technology and new methods of treatment have greatly changed the demands on all health professionals. Competent health professionals are characterized not only by their professional capabilities, but by how effectively they can mobilize the resources available to manage a patient's care. Such effective mobilization requires a redefinition and reinterpretation of professional boundaries.

REFERENCES

Abramson, Marcia and Black, Rita Beck: Extending the boundaries of life: Implications for practice. *Health and Social Work, 10:* 165–173, 1985.

Achenbaum, W. Andrew and Levin, Jeffrey S.: What does gerontology mean? *The Gerontologist, 29,* 393–400, 1989.

American Medical Association, Task Force for the Evaluation of Experimental Programs for Developing the Registered Care Technician. Personal communication, 1989.

Boettcher, Elaine Grace: Boundary marking: A social ecological study of human need satisfaction among institutionalized elderly persons. *Journal of Psychosocial Nursing and Mental Health Services, 23:* 25–30, 1985.

Brown, L. David: *Managing Conflict at Organizational Interfaces.* Reading, Addison-Wesley, 1983.

Bruhn, John G.: Occupational therapy in the 21st century: An outsider's view. *American Journal of Occupational Therapy, 45:* 775–780, 1991.

Bureau of Allied Health Manpower: *Education for the Allied Health Professions and Services: Report of the Allied Health Professions Education Subcommittee of the National Advisory Health Council.* Washington, U.S. Government Printing Office, 1967.

Colman, Wendy: Maintaining autonomy: The struggle between occupational therapy and physical medicine. *The American Journal of Occupational Therapy, 46:* 63–70, 1992.

Colwill, Jack M.: Where have all the primary care applicants gone? *New England Journal of Medicine, 326:* 387–383, 1992.

Eaton, Gail and Webb, Barbara: Boundary encroachment: Pharmacists in the clinical setting. *Sociology of Health and Illness, 1:* 69–89, 1979.

Fagin, Claire M.: Collaboration between nurses and physicians: No longer a choice. *Academic Medicine, 67:* 295–303, 1992.

Fein, Rashi: *Medical Care, Medical Costs: The Search for a Health Insurance Policy.* Cambridge, Harvard University Press, 1986.

Freddi, Giorgi: Problems in organizational rationality in health systems: Political controls and policy options. In Freddi, Giorgio and Bjorkman, James W. (eds.): *Controlling Medical Professionals: The Comparative Politics of Health Governance.* CA, Sage, 1989.

Freidson, Eliot: *Doctoring Together: A Study of Professional Social Control.* New York, Elsevier, 1975.

Fuchs, Victor R. *The Health Economy.* Cambridge, Harvard University Press, 1986.

Ginzberg, Eli: *Health Manpower and Health Policy.* Montclair, Allanheld, Osmun and Company, 1978.

Gitterman, Alex: Testing professional authority and boundaries. *Social Casework: The Journal of Contemporary Social Work, 70:* 165–171, 1989.

Haddad, Amy Marie: The boundaries of beneficence: Ethical obligations and the noncompliant client. *Pride Institute Journal of Long Term Home Health Care, 8:* 19–23, 1989.

Hankin, Robert A. Turf wars. *Dental Management, 29:* 17–19, 1989.

Humphrey, Carolyn Joy: The home as a setting for care: Clarifying the boundaries of practice. *Nursing Clinics of North America, 23:* 305–314, 1988.

Institute of Medicine: *Allied Health Services: Avoiding Crises.* Washington, National Academy Press, 1989.

Jonas, Steven: *Medical Mystery.* New York, W.W. Norton, 1978.

Kaufman, Sharon R. and Becker, Gaylene: Content and boundaries of medicine in long-term care: Physicians talk about stroke. *The Gerontologist, 31:* 238–245, 1991.

Kronus, Carol L.: The evolution of occupational power: An historical study of task boundaries between physicians and pharmacists. *Sociology of Work and Occupations, 3:* 3–37, 1976.

Lessnoff-Caravaglia, Gari: *Health Care of the Elderly.* New York, Human Sciences Press, 1980.

Mauksch, Ingeborg G. The nurse practitioner movement—where does it go from here? *American Journal of Public Health, 68:* 1074–1075, 1978.

Morganstein, Warren M.: Auxiliary personnel in dentistry: An epoch of turf, trends, and territoriality. *American Journal of Hospital Pharmacy, 46:* 507–514, 1989.

National Commission on Allied Health Education: *The Future of Allied Health Education: New Alliances for the 1980's.* San Francisco, Jossey-Bass, 1980.

Norman, Geoffrey R.: Defining competence: A methodological review. In Neufeld, Victor R. and Norman, Geoffrey R. (eds.): *Assessing Clinical Competence.* New York, Springer, 1985.

Overholser, James C. and Fine, Mark A.: Defining the boundaries of professional competence: Managing subtle cases of clinical incompetence. *Professional Practice: Research and Practice, 21:* 462–469, 1990.

Pritchard, Peter: Managing the world outside the practice. *The Practitioner, 233:* 905–907, 1989.

Reich, Warren T. (ed.): *Encyclopedia of Bioethics.* Vol. 3. New York, Macmillan, 1978.

Ritchey, Ferris J., Pinkston, Dorothy, Goldbaum, Joanne E. and Heerten, Margret E.: Perceptual correlates of physician referral to physical therapists: Implications for role expansion. *Social Science and Medicine, 28:* 69–80, 1989.

Rose, Marion H. and Killien, Marcia: Risk and vulnerability: A case for differentiation. *Advances in Nursing Science, 4:* 60–73, 1983.

Scott, Anne L.: Human interaction and personal boundaries. *Journal of Psychosocial Nursing, 26:* 23–27, 1988.

Segal, Erich: *Doctors.* New York, Bantam Books, 1988.

Serrett, Karen Diasio: Another look at occupational therapy's history: Paradigm or pair-of-hands? *Occupational Therapy in Mental Health, 5:* 1–32, 1985.

Stone, Michael H.: Boundary violations between therapist and patient. *Psychiatric Annals, 6:* 8–21, 1976.

Trier, William C.: Evaluation and treatment planning for patients with cleft lip and cleft palate. *Clinics in Plastic Surgery, 12(4):* 553–572, October 1985.

Uzych, Leo: Pharmacists and the right to prescribe: Ugly "Turf" battle or opportunity for improved patient care. *Florida M.A., 75:* 143–144, 1988.

Westra, Bonnie: Winning hearts and minds: Let's hold on to our own. *Nursing, 16:* 52–53, 1986.

Yerxa, Elizabeth J.: Occupational therapy: An endangered species or an academic discipline in 21st century? *The American Journal of Occupational Therapy, 45:* 680–685, 1991.

Chapter 4

INTERACTIONS BETWEEN
BOUNDARIES AND PERSONALITY

Today's manager is a "change manager" in a society that
may be described as overtly dependent on and fixated with
technology and high rates of change. Therefore, the manager must develop his skills and insights to manage change
while influencing its rate, direction and extent. The path
for developing these skills, awareness, and insights lies
within oneself.

Bob Messing
The Tao of Management, *1989, p. viii*

Donald T. Phillips (1992), in his analytical study of Abraham Lincoln
as a leader, notes how effective Lincoln was as a manager of
boundaries. He aimed at the "elevation of men" and especially lashed
out at the institution of slavery. By vehemently opposing slavery, Lincoln was able to mobilize his followers in a common mission. Had
Lincoln not been the leader he was, secession, in 1860, could have led to
the further partitioning of the country into an infinite number of smaller,
separate pieces, some retaining slavery, some not (pp. 172–173).

In the health arena, we have had a leader, who, during the past
decade, has helped to cross boundaries with respect to smoking and
AIDS. C. Everett Koop, as Surgeon General, not only crossed the conservative boundaries of his boss, but chose to take on topics that crossed
sensitive economic boundaries with tobacco companies and the varying
moral boundaries regarding sexual behavior of the general population.
Smoking in public places, discouraged in earlier years, now is illegal in
many cities. Sexual behavior, which was discussed in privacy, now is
explicitly and publicly debated.

People who tackle issues that cross boundaries are not only brave, but
must exert strong leadership if they are to be listened to and, eventually,
successful. At the level of the organization, the act of defining a mission
and protecting its integrity is managing a boundary. At the level of the

individual, leadership entails managing the complex transactions between the leader and the led (Gilmore, 1982). While much of the leadership research has focused on the leader-follower relationship, the emergent task of leadership is also the creation and maintenance of an environment in which people can be productive.

Leadership: Styles and Tasks

Studies and theories of leadership may be divided into three groups. The first group treats leadership primarily as a function of the personality of the leader, of inborn traits or traits developed early in life. This is the "great man" school or *trait approach,* which seems outdated for a world in which the influencers and the leaders must often negotiate and mediate in order to lead rather than to play out their basic personalities. Yet, many organizations are still largely shaped by the personality of the leader (Sheldon, 1975).

The second group believes that leadership is a *personal-behavioral* function of the interaction of the leader and those whom he leads. In this view, effective leadership is a function of the fit of personality with the expectations and personality characteristics of subordinates and group needs. Blake and Mouton's grid (1969) and Tannenbaum and Schmidt's (1973) boss-subordinate approaches are both of this kind. Each allows the leader to characterize managerial style along specified dimensions.

The third group of leadership theories is based on the *situation model.* Schein (1972) posits that the leader must diagnose the people, tasks, groups, organizational structure and environment, in order to choose appropriate behavior to lead. The situation dictates the required behavior subject to modification by the leader's predilections. Fiedler's (1967) research has found, for example, that task-oriented leadership is best under very favorable or very unfavorable situations, but person-oriented leadership is best for in-between situations.

Leaders must scan and span (manage) and review the boundaries between the organization and its environments, external and internal, for trends, fit, and problems. The complexity of modern organizations is such that most decisions cannot be made by a single leader. The decisions are interdependent both with other managers within the organization and with other decision makers outside the organization.

Sheldon (1975) says that managership is the solving of today's problems, while leadership is the identification of tomorrow's problems and the setting in place of problem solving mechanisms needed today. The top manager must be able to manage tasks and people but also reexamine boundaries (actual and ideological) and review organizational mechanisms in light of environmental change. Sheldon presents several case studies to illustrate how boundaries are managed in a variety of health care settings, e.g., hospital mergers, establishing a "problem-based" curriculum in a medical school, and restructuring nursing services in a hospital.

The personalities of leader-managers are intimately related to their style of decision-making. A variety of labels come to mind—logical/ nonlogical, objective/subjective, toughminded/softheaded, analytic/ synthetic, scientific/artistic, and reasoning/intuiting. People have these characteristics in varying degrees and combinations. These personality characteristics blend with a person's values and beliefs in making decisions. Given different values and beliefs, one manager may recognize a problem in a particular situation while another may not. The identification of relevant and appropriate alternatives depends on individual value systems (Kast and Rosenzweig, 1985).

Boundary disputes usually involve disputes between values and beliefs. Beliefs are predictive judgments. They are convictions that certain things are true or real. An individual's system of beliefs is accumulated over time and adjusted continually according to experience and observation. Both values and beliefs are important in influencing managerial decision-making. Values and beliefs, along with personality characteristics, e.g., flexibility and control, influence how a manager will assess a boundary situation and the types of options that will be perceived in a situation of boundary conflict. How managers manage their values and beliefs and those of their coworkers is the key to successful boundary management. For example, a manager might be confronted with the following situation:

The head of Department A asks for more space to relieve the current crowded working quarters of his employees. The Department head appeals to the manager to give him space that is nearby and vacant, but which is being held by the manager for a new operation planned in the immediate future. The manager agrees to give Department A the space on a temporary basis and both parties put their agreement in writing. Several months later, the manager notices that the space he loaned to Department A is being remodeled and that it is to house new and expanded departmental functions rather than relieve the existing crowded conditions of Department A as its head had indicated.

While this boundary issue obviously involves the breach of an agreement, its resolution involves the manager's values and beliefs. The manager could, at one extreme, stop the remodeling and "take back" the space because it is being used differently than was agreed upon. At the opposite extreme, the manager could let the situation pass until he actually needs the space for the new operation. Space means power and status. Once space is acquired, it is seldom relinquished, it must be taken away. Space is so prized, it is often obtained deviously or under false pretenses. Those who control space have power. If the manager delays confronting the department head about the "misuse" of space, it is likely that by the time the manager needs the space for a new operation, the department head will be able to justify retaining the space. On the other hand, if the manager confronts the department head immediately, and takes back the space, the confrontation will involve the value and belief systems of both parties—not the space, but what was right and wrong about how the space was acquired, and how it is being used, will be the major issue. Considering the disruption that would result from overt action, most managers would accept the *fait accompli;* however, they would be very cautious about releasing future space.

Such a situation, in the long run, can result in suspicion and lack of cooperation, which can permeate an institution. Cooperation depends, to a large extent, on trust. The manager who uses inappropriate tactics to obtain resources may win in the short run, but, in the long run, the failure to live up to agreements will damage everyone. The chief executives responsible for both managers may wash their hands of the affair, letting their subordinates fight it out. Business and government organizations sometimes act as though fundamental values, such as trust, honesty, and fairness, are obsolete and success in the "real world" requires ruthlessness and single minded devotion to one's goals. In the long run, however, organizations existing in such an atmosphere will find it impossible to generate the internal esprit de corps to succeed.

Values and Boundaries

Human beings hold two kinds of theories of action. The first is their espoused theory, which is composed of beliefs, values, and attitudes. The second is their theory-in-use, which is the one they actually use when they act (Argyris, 1990). The zeal with which we defend our boundaries is a good indication of how much we value something when it is threatened.

New facts and information are unlikely to change the intensity of our defense. We change our behavior only when we believe that change will be of significant value (benefit) to us and that the costs and risks associated with that change will be acceptable. Thus, we may modify the values, beliefs and attitudes we espouse (our social virtues) when they have direct, perceivable benefits to us. The interplay between the social virtues we espouse and the realities we perceive constitutes personality. Personality is not so much who we are as it is how we act on our perceived realities. For example, we may say that honesty is the best policy, but we tend to practice defensive honesty. The house-seller asks more money than he expects to receive because he knows the buyer will offer less than he expects to pay.

In organizations that are genuinely concerned with people, individuals may find themselves in a dilemma, espousing values that are difficult to implement. For example, management may espouse excellence, yet mediocrity exists unless it is continually held in check. Or, management may espouse employee involvement, yet many employees distance themselves from becoming responsible for imputing new ideas into the organization. These discrepancies create what Argyris calls organizational defensiveness. To overcome this defensiveness, Argyris suggests a new theory-in-use or a commitment to new social virtues. These virtues are to increase employees' capacity to confront their own ideas, to advocate their positions, to encourage employees to say what they know, yet fear to say, to advocate their principles, values, and beliefs that encourage others to do the same, and to create in employees, self-reflection and self-examination.

Argyris notes that many managers are concerned with control and maintain rigid boundaries in attempts to ensure their own success. Yet, in situations of managerial tight control, managers often develop their own boundaries and pay more attention to their own well-being than to the organization as a whole. Employees in such a situation may lose their sense of accountability or initiative. Different consequences follow from the control and commitment models. The first consequence of the control model is consistent with unilateral control, power with position, the manipulation of people through activities, and the private evaluation of individual performance. On the other hand, the commitment model emphasizes bilateral control and mutuality, power with expertise, the motivation of people through internal commitment, and the public testing of performance evaluations. The control model encourages the values of win/don't lose. The commitment model encourages the values of winning together/it's o.k. to fail (Blake and Mouton, 1961).

The Issue of Control

In order to implement these new social virtues, a manager has to be willing to relinquish some control, to share responsibility with employees. Webster's definition of "control" is "to exercise restraint or direction over; to hold back or in check." Control often possesses a negative connotation, implying that without control, people would be irresponsible and would misuse or deplete material resources, and that someone is needed to hold irrational behavior in check and keep an organization focused on its goals. Control over resources, however, is not the only factor that determines the direction of an organization. Managers who are given the function of control have their own needs to satisfy, and this influences the ways in which they use control. Personality plays a large role in management style and, hence, in how managers use their control (Bruhn, 1991; Bruhn, 1993).

Control, Trust, and Creativity

According to Bennis and Nanus (1985), trust is the lubrication that allows organizations to work. Trust implies accountability, predictability, and reliability. We trust people who are predictable and whose positions are known. Managers who trust employees are less controlling and are more likely to delegate authority than managers who are distrustful. Distrustful managers are less likely to be accessible to employees because they have full appointment schedules and are always busy monitoring the work of employees. Such managers have only a day-to-day perspective of their organization; their schedules do not permit time to plan, reflect, or evaluate. Distrustful and controlling managers are at risk for burnout or other health problems because they "live their jobs in detail." They have no time to lead or to promote their own professional growth or that of others. The following illustration makes this point:

The Dean of a large college on a university campus was energetic and positive, and was seen as a strong leader, both within and outside the college. The Dean had an Associate Dean and two Assistant Deans, but delegated minimally. The Associate Dean was given responsibility for advising students and keeping the bulletin boards current. The Assistant

Deans advised students and handled academic grievances. The Dean retained all authority and responsibility for the college curriculum, budget, space, equipment, and personnel. The Dean worked at his job intensely and told his subordinates very little. After two years in the job, the Dean experienced chest pain and other cardiac symptoms and was told by his physician to "slow down." He did not perceive that the *way* he worked was a problem, only how *long* he worked. He dismissed his Associate Dean, claiming he did little. His two Assistant Deans chose to return to the classroom.

The Dynamics of Management Style

We have discussed the interplay between four components of management style: personality, control, trust, and creativity. No single combination of these factors makes a good manager. The dynamics—how managers use personality and their attitudes and feelings about control, trust, and creativity—distinguish effective from ineffective managers. The emotional aspect of managerial behavior is as important as the intellectual or rational aspect in determining who will be an effective manager. Effective managers are good at managing values—the organization's, their employees', and their own. Effective managers seek ways to create an environment that will maximize values and achieve desired outcomes. An excessively controlling manager who puts the personal values of power and prestige above the values of the organization and its employees will not create an environment that will satisfy other people's values. If work morale and productivity decline, the manager may become even more controlling to ensure that his or her values are satisfied. The opposite situation exists for the indecisive manager; in the absence of decisions, employees often take on responsibility for decision making to satisfy their values (Bruhn, 1990).

Controlling, distrustful managers inhibit organizational creativity. Without some degree of trust, employees cannot experience the autonomy needed to be creative. As a consequence of excessive control and distrust, employees can become submissive ("yes men") or silent, dissatisfied, and critical.

Managerial Personalities

There are as many styles of management as there are personalities. Despite variations in personality, the elements of control, trust, and creativity exist in varying degrees in all managers and affect how they manage. We tend to type managers as we do other people. Typing has its dangers, however. Typing is sometimes limited to single traits, which are then labeled as good or bad; if types are generalized, they can be detrimental to the recipient of the label. Bureaucracies tend to type people to fit the requirements of their hierarchies (e.g., teachers type students, police type criminals, physicians type patients, and managers type employees). On the positive side, typing can be a means to help understand people better. Types are often ideals, and no individual fits a type exactly; most people are a mixture of types.

Several writers in the area of leadership have grouped managers according to the values they exhibit as they manage. The values a manager holds will influence, directly or indirectly, all of his or her decisions and, in turn, the character and direction of the organization. Jennings (1960) described four groups of managers based on their values: The *prince* seeks power and is concerned with establishing a reputation and perpetuating an image. The *hero* is a serious, dedicated, intuitive leader who pursues a specific purpose and has a deep sense of mission. The *superman* stands for excellence. Jennings notes that all leaders have a mixture of the prince, the hero, and superman. The *team man* is a relatively new type of manager who emphasizes cooperation and teamsmanship in completing tasks.

In an extensive study of 250 managers from 12 major companies in different parts of the United States, Maccoby (1976) also found four types of managers. The *craftsman* holds traditional values of the work ethic, respect for people, a concern for quality and thrift, and an enjoyment of building. The *jungle fighter's* goal is power. Jungle fighters tend to see their peers as accomplices or enemies and their subordinates as objects to be utilized. The *company man's* strongest traits are his concern with the human side of his company and his commitment to maintaining the organization's integrity. The *gamesman's* main interest is in challenge and competitive activity, in which he can prove himself a winner. He responds to work and life as a game.

Garfield (1986) and Ouchi (1981) discuss Theory Z, a management style that blends Japanese and American traits. From Japan, for example, the theory borrows long-term employment, consensual decision making, slow promotion and evaluation, and concern for the whole; from America, informal types of control, specialized career paths, and individual achievement. Type Z companies are known for high morale, low turnover, and company loyalty. According to Theory Z, the way to sustain higher levels of production is to assume that workers have "higher needs" for self-esteem, want to belong to an organization of which they can be proud, and want autonomy and responsibility at work.

Victims of Management Style

Excessively controlling managers can create anger and hostility among employees who may, in some circumstances, feel their rights are being infringed on and who may file grievances. Controlling managers are more concerned with the growth of resources and products than with the growth of employees. Hence, employees may be transferred according to the needs of the organization without regard to how the transfers will benefit them. The manager who cultivates employees to excess can also produce victims. Employees can become overly dependent on supervisors for advice, guidance, and, in some cases, for making career decisions for them. All managerial styles in their exaggerated forms create victims.

Employees are not always in a position to choose their managers. Indeed, changes in managers and management style have been the reason some employees take early retirement, seek transfers, or terminate employment. How employees adapt to a manager's style is an individual matter. Different personalities, especially in people who are in positions of authority, arouse different conscious and unconscious feelings in employees regarding authority, power, and parenting. Management style can profoundly influence the progression of an employee's career. Sometimes the only preventive action an employee can take to avoid an open conflict with a manager and the related risk to his future with the organization is to leave. Managers are unlikely to alter their styles; they have reached their managerial positions by being the kinds of people they are, and they may not be fully aware of how their managerial behavior affects others.

Team Managers and Creative Gamesmen

The complexities of the work world, and of management, make it difficult to be an effective manager if one's scope of concern is limited to isolated segments of the work situation. It is no longer efficient or sufficient to focus only on salary and benefits, job skills, or quality. A more global perspective that includes all of these factors is needed. Some people refer to this perspective as systems thinking; whatever it is labeled, it acknowledges that the times change the work environment, and that all aspects of work and the work environment have an interacting and reinforcing effect on each other. For example, the world of the 90's is putting unprecedented pressures on managers in health care fields. When Medicare and Medicaid were passed, hospitals and health professions schools experienced enormous pressures to expand. Then the pressures changed, much hospital space was deemed surplus, and concerns were expressed about an "oversupply of health professionals." Because of generous reimbursement formulas for subspecialists, power within the health professions moved toward them. However, current trends indicate a coming revival of generalist training and generalist influence.

Managers must have a broad view, must anticipate and create changes, and must direct the effects as much as possible by addressing the different and changing needs of workers. Health professions managers and leaders must prepare their institutions for new sets of priorities. Managing is like directing an orchestra.

Landau and Stout (1979) point out that we are often told that "to manage is to control," as if all a good manager has to do is to learn a set of control procedures and ensure that these are complied with. Contrary to the proverb, the ability to control and the necessity to manage have an inverse relationship. Management is an experimental process, the point of which is to discover that knowledge which eventually permits control.

Maccoby (1976) talks about the creative gamesman manager. The gamesman's values include a concern for people. The creative gamesman manager is concerned about how well he or she develops followers to become leaders themselves. Three key traits of the gamesman are:

1. an ability to see the whole and not merely the parts,
2. the ability to create an environment in which others work better, and
3. the ability to understand other people's weaknesses and strengths in terms of the job requirements for the group.

In studies of managers and workers, it has been found that different types of people have different values and needs. A work environment that fits or encourages one managerial type may be frustrating for another. In the final analysis, what matters is how well the manager and worker adapt to each other and to the rest of organization for which they work.

Compromises to Control

Pascale (1990) has likened the control-commitment models of Argyris to hard minds versus soft hearts. Hard minds pertains to a bottom-line orientation. A hard-minded emphasis all too often spawns a short-term focus, and fosters organizations that treat their employees like robots. At the other extreme, preoccupation with soft-hearted values can lead to wastefulness and the loss of efficiency. There is an essential tension between hard minds and soft hearts. Hard-minded executives are tied to goals that are unambiguous and quantifiable. In contrast, soft-hearted values pertain to intangibles that are tied to higher order ideas affecting employees.

The hard minds/soft hearts dichotomy challenges companies to be caring, yet engender realism. One of its pitfalls is that companies overreach. They set themselves up to charges of hypocrisy when they get tough and the company's behavior doesn't square with its espoused values. Pascale proposes a new mindset that embraces this paradox, that of shared values. He uses Honda as the quintessential example of a learning organization. Virtually all of Honda's top executives share the view that all learning comes from values. Employees at all levels of Honda report that Honda's values are brought to bear once or twice a week in determining how a particular problem should be solved, or how a person should be treated. It is the everyday acknowledgement and continuity of these values that generate trust. Values and trust establish the preconditions that encourage individuals to think, experiment, and improve. Once enduring values, trust, and empowerment are in place, an organization can begin to learn.

Harrington (1985) advocates the need for managerial strategic flexibility. She notes that many companies put themselves into strategic groups in terms of which customer they will serve and how they will compete. Guerrilla strategies define boundaries rigidly for purposes of market competition. Harrington's view is that these aggressive strategies carry over into managerial problem-solving within the company. The way managers conceptualize their market and means of competing, sets the stage for employee autonomy and risk-taking. Forces, such as shorter product lives, are blurring industry boundaries and must be translated into new ways of doing things. This provides the opportunity for companies to become more flexible and innovative with respect to the management of a more team-oriented labor force.

The management of boundaries is the management of people's personalities and perceptions. Personality develops over the course of an individual's life and influences the person's perception of reality and behavior in organizations. Organizations can only be as creative and adaptive as the people they employ.

Research has suggested that various traits interact to form different personality types. Examples are: 1) the *authoritarian* personality, which is characterized by rigidity, obedience, submission to authority, and a tendency to stereotype; 2) the *Machiavellian* personality, which is oriented toward manipulation and control, with a low sensitivity to others, and 3) the *existential* personality, which tends to place a high value on choice, attempts to maintain an accurate perception of reality, and tries to understand other people (Adorno, Frenkel-Brunswik, Levinson and Sanford, 1950; Brown, 1965; Siegel, 1973; Gemmill and Heisler, 1972, Kelly, 1980). Personality acts as a perceptual filter through which we see the world.

Perhaps the most significant illustration of the effect of personality in organizational life is found in research that has drawn parallels between common neurotic styles of behavior and common modes of organizational failure (Kets De Vries and Miller, 1986; Miller and Friesen, 1984; Miller, Kets De Vries and Toulouse, 1982). Stagnant bureaucracies are exemplified by organizations that lack clear goals, lack initiative, react sluggishly to environmental change, and are pervaded by managerial apathy, frustration, and inaction. On an individual level, the depressive personality style exhibits similar features. All people develop behavior patterns for dealing with their environment that are deeply embedded, pervasive, and likely to continue; the personal behavior of its administrators shapes the way in which an organization adapts to its environment. In an organization where power is broadly distributed, the culture and structure is determined by many managers, and the relationship between personality and organizational style is tenuous. However, in those organizations in which power is concentrated, an extreme style at the top of the organization can impact all levels.

Available evidence seems to indicate that no personality traits or characteristics consistently distinguish a leader from his followers. There is some evidence, however, that a leader, if he is to be followed, probably cannot be markedly different from his subordinates (Spotts, 1969).

A number of studies indicate that leadership does not occur in a vacuum, but at a particular time and place and under a particular set of circumstances. Therefore, a given situation determines, to some degree, the kinds of leadership skills and behavior that may be required. Different leadership styles help particular groups to function more effectively. For example, democratic or participative leadership behavior tends to be associated with productivity and increased worker morale. Directive leadership, which has been found to lead to high productivity, often results in low morale and commitment to work. Different leadership practices seem appropriate for different situations.

A growing body of research indicates clear differences between the behavior of high and low production workers in real life situations. The quality of the leader-subordinate relationship (the degree of respect and consideration the leader shows for the worker's needs) appears to be a crucial factor. Employee-centered leadership tends to be more closely associated with productivity, morale, and job satisfaction than does production-centered leadership. Leaders accomplish their work through other people, and their success as leaders depends upon their ability to enlist and maintain follower commitment and collaboration for the attainment of organizational goals (Spotts, 1969).

Blake and Mouton (1985) point out that whenever leaders approach a situation, they act on subjective appraisal, which may or may not be close to objective reality. We act on our assumptions, which become part of our beliefs and attitudes. These assumptions guide our behavior. They constitute our personal leadership styles. Leaders seldom verbalize their assumptions, but they do act on them. Therefore, it is important to understand a leader's assumptions.

We have discussed various personality characteristics and their relationship to management styles and the management of boundaries. We have assumed that leaders lead and managers manage. Both leaders and managers should be involved in boundary management. Leaders must be concerned with boundaries as they plan for change; managers must manage the accommodations that must be made to boundaries in response to change. Organizations with leaders who do not manage boundaries effectively usually replace them after it becomes apparent that the organization is adrift or is soon to meet its demise. Managers who cannot manage boundary conflicts are also a liability to an organization.

Leaders who are ineffective in managing boundaries are characterized by buck passing, unwillingness to make decisions, and/or isolation from subordinates. Decisions eventually have to be made; if they are not made directly by the leader, they will be made by others in the organization or by events. Sometimes, organizations select a compromising leader who is not effective in managing boundaries, especially when the organization has experienced a period of turmoil and change, or is attempting to cope with warring interest groups. Abdication of the powers of leadership is, itself, a type of management style, and is often linked with such personality traits as wanting to be liked by others and an inability to cope with conflict.

Kets de Vries and Miller (1984) note that managers may victimize subordinates by indecisiveness. Victimization has long-term effects on an organization. Employees find it difficult to grow professionally; they see themselves as expendable. Indecisive managers often believe they have to take some action while contemplating a final decision. Interim decisions are often more destructive than deferral of action until a final decision has been made.

Indecisive managers have little time for management. As Oncken and Wass (1974) point out, many indecisive managers have too many monkeys on their backs; they do not have control over the timing and content of what they do. The monkey-on-the-back analogy refers to the need to transfer the initiative from the manager's back to that of his or her subordinates. If managers are indecisive, they keep the initiative and accumulate the problems of subordinates. Managers will, in turn, have less time to make decisions, encouraging their indecisiveness.

Indecisive managers relinquish or pass out of their socially-defined roles (Hill *et al.*, 1979). They are easy targets for burnout due to an over-accumulation of monkeys on their backs or to hearing loss caused by the persistent loud chattering of monkeys who are trying to make decisions for management. Zoo keepers need to be carefully chosen for their management styles. Some managers let the monkeys run at will, some severely restrict the movement of the monkeys, and others coexist with the monkeys. Indecisive managers often let the monkeys run at will, tolerating a variety of monkey business that may be destructive to the organization.

Indecisive managers may attempt to make their employees happier; the manager may believe that he or she is not doing enough for the employees, and is thereby causing their disruptive behavior. Indecisive managers frequently are people who have a great need to be liked; hence, they may interpret monkey business as evidence that they have failed. The root cause of their difficulties, their management styles, are so tied up with their good intentions that criticism of their styles could be taken as personal criticism. Hence, it is difficult for indecisive managers to prevent or correct monkey business without outside intervention. Unfortunately, the need for outside consultation usually is not recognized by the manager, and sometimes not by the manager's supervisor, until the monkeys have taken over the zoo and pandemonium reigns (Bruhn, 1990).

Indecisiveness is a way of abdicating leadership. When leaders abdicate, lower level employees are forced to resolve issues. Lacking the knowledge to guide their choices, lower level employees typically face opposing choices: to burrow more deeply into their work, or to exert pressure to fill the leadership void and attempt to allay their anxieties through monkey business. Organizations with poorly drawn boundaries are most susceptible to monkey business.

The establishment of clear boundaries does not imply that leaders should be authoritarian. Rather, boundaries help employees to interpret and understand what is real and what is illusionary behavior, what is permissible and what is not, and what are and are not appropriate ways to express opinions. When boundaries are official, workers feel authorized to work. Perhaps more important, boundaries help manage the interdependencies among workers and between workers and managers in complex organizations.

Monkey business tends to erupt in situations of stress or uncertainty. For example, problems will occur when there is a change in managers, especially when accompanied by a dramatic shift in management style; when the goals of the work unit and the organization are not clear, or the goals of one are perceived to have changed and are out of place with the other; when there has been a substantial turnover of employees in a short period of time; when the demand for the product or service produced by the work unit decreases and a replacement has not yet been clearly formulated; when employees' jobs have become so specialized that they do not feel or see how they contribute to the whole or the final product; and when there is little or no opportunity to critique the process or product of the work unit.

Monkey business is based on the psychology of projecting the bad on others. Monkey business helps us to contain our anxiety. Monkey business helps us to register our protests against a manager. Management style can facilitate monkey business, but is not the sole cause of it.

Closely related to the notion of personality is self concept, the way we see ourselves. Each of us has a self-image that influences what we say, do, or perceive about the world. This image acts as a filter that screens out certain things and provides an idiosyncratic flavor to our behavior. Our self concept is composed of four interacting factors: values, beliefs, competencies, and personal goals. We try to maintain our images of ourselves by engaging in behaviors that are consistent with our values, beliefs, competencies, and goals. How managers see themselves influences how they react to others. It is important to be aware of the different ways in which we distort and bias information about other people, events, and objects so we can be more effective in our dealings with others. The well-known theorem of the sociologist, W.I. Thomas (Volkart, 1951), is, situations that are perceived to be real are real in their consequences.

Boundaries of Self-Control

The concept of perceived personal control has received a great deal of attention over the past decade or so. In general, increasing the perception that one is in control of one's destiny has been found to have positive effects, whereas decreasing the amount of perceived personal control has been associated with negative effects. For example, increased control has been identified as beneficial in dealing with stress, coping with diversity, adjusting to a home for the aged, learning new material, and succeeding in a weight-loss program. On the other hand, a perceived decline in one's ability to control a situation has been tied to feelings of crowding and to learned helplessness and depression (Burger, McWard and La Tolle, 1989).

However, people sometimes do not prefer to be in control or react to increased control over them with negative effect. Paradoxically, people want to feel in control of their destinies, yet they often freely relinquish that control.

Exercising control can lead to feelings of competency and mastery and can help to overcome or avoid feelings of helplessness (Seligman, 1975). Although obtaining control over an event or project often means an increased opportunity to make things turn out the way we want, this is not always the case. Miller's (1980) "mini-max" hypothesis is relevant here. She has argued that people facing potentially aversive consequences select the option that ensures that they will experience aversive stimuli within a range they find tolerable. People are said to relinquish control to others when such action increases their chances of staying within their range of tolerance.

Health care programming and policy, in the 1990's, are largely shaped by financing and increased corporate control. In this environment, hospital pharmacy managers face new challenges in their ability to tolerate ambiguity that comes from relating to a hospital's corporate administration on one hand and the professional staff and patients on the other (Pierpaoli, 1987). A director of pharmacy faces two distinct categories of ambiguity: those that are rooted in issues and matters external to the pharmacy department, and those that are internal to the department. Extradepartmental sources of ambiguity include structural or organizational barriers that distort power and authority. The pharmacy director must be a spanner of boundaries because the support of both medical and hospital administrators is required to make changes in drug-use policy. Power and influence is in a constant state of flux between these two constituencies. Interpersonal role conflict and ambiguity can also exist between directors of pharmacy and third-tier hospital administrators. Ambiguity and conflict can stem from the superimposition on pharmacy clinical practice systems of rigid rules and regulations of professional and hospital licensing bodies or standards of accrediting agencies. In their quest to achieve greater professionalization, hospital pharmacists have expanded their roles as patient advocates in drug therapy and now operate in areas typically occupied by other health professions. In addition, pharmacy has been preoccupied with the evaluation of pharmacy intervention in the hospital setting.

In attempting to garner more staff and resources for expanding clinical pharmaceutical services, a director of pharmacy is faced with questions of efficiency and cost-containment. Interdepartmental forces also create uncertainty and ambiguity for hospital pharmacy program managers. These include clinical specialists and other pharmacists who perform purely dispensing roles without opportunities for professional advancement and technicians whose missions and roles have not been identified or integrated into the discipline of pharmacy (Pierpaoli, 1987).

The forces impacting upon pharmacy from outside its boundaries give it a low degree of control and a high level of ambiguity. It has been shown that when rewards become more external to the individual, perceived ambiguity and conflict increase (Dailey, 1979). Cohesive groups tend to buffer individual members from perceived ambiguity and help reduce anxiety and tension among members. It appears that pharmacy has sacrificed group cohesion in its attempt to broaden its boundaries. These broadened boundaries provide an opportunity for a greater variety of pharmacy-related workers and technicians to enter the pharmacy workforce. This heterogeneity helps to lessen the degree of control over the profession of pharmacy. These internal changes, along with the tact, diplomacy, vision and creative skill needed for dealing with a variety of constituencies, have made pharmacy a profession in transition. The issue of control, as discussed earlier, lies largely with players outside of pharmacy.

As Harris and Dewey (1984, p. 390) explained, " . . . boundary persons frequently feel responsible for and responsive to people and things they cannot control. They frequently report qualitative underload and quantitative overload, as well as social isolation. The incidence of disease is significantly higher in people in boundary positions, such as salespeople and administrators, than it is in people whose roles are inside the organization."

Territoriality and Stress

French and Caplan (1970), in a study of the impact of organizational territory on engineers working in an administrative unit and, conversely, administrators working in an engineering unit, concluded that territoriality is a powerful stressor. They found that men working in alien territories experienced stress, and they concluded that crossing an organizational boundary and working in an alien territory entails stress and strain and poses a threat to one's health.

Organizational territoriality and accompanying possessiveness seem to develop around parts of the organization that have become familiar. Thus, stress frequently increases when one leaves the home base. An exception occurs when individuals seek refuge in another area to escape temporary stressors in their home territory. The managerial implication of the territory stressor is that managerially initiated changes of familiar patterns can trigger significant stress. Even if a person stays in his or her own territory, this stressor can be a factor when other groups enter the territory (Ivancevich and Matteson, 1980).

Stress and Personality in Organizations

Few well-designed studies include personality measures with organizational dimensions. One important determination is the primary source of reported stress: is it the job itself, the personality of the worker, or the fit between the two which causes the stress? A second problem evolves around the traditional measures of stress. Most organizational research either uses a paper and pencil measure of stress or assumes role stress to be a proxy measure. Several researchers have argued for the use of physiologic stress measures. Frew and Bruning (1987), when they studied the relationship between perceived organizational variables (sources of role stress and job characteristics), personality variables (manifest needs, Type A personality [hard driving, impatient types], and self-esteem), physiological measures (blood pressure, pulse rate and galvanic skin response), and attitudinal measures of stress, found that personality accounted for a significant contribution to manifest anxiety and job characteristics were related to diastolic blood pressure.

Caplan and Jones (1975) found that job involvement and characteristic Type A personality is both a blessing and a curse. The higher the status of people's occupations, the more involved they were in their work. Highly involved persons obtained great emotional rewards from their successes, but paid a great psychological price when they faced the prospect of failure in their work roles.

A group of managers classed as either Type A or Type B (relaxed, less time-bound than Type A) was studied to examine the effects of job satisfaction as a moderator between a common job stressor (role ambiguity) and several coronary indicators. For Type A individuals, the results supported the hypothesis that changes in ambiguity are associated with changes in blood pressure and that intrinsic job satisfaction appeared to have both a direct and indirect moderating effect on these changes. For Type B individuals, the effects on blood pressure were the opposite, indicating that individuals who are characteristically Types A and B may "fit" their environments differently (Howard, Cunningham & Rechnitzer, 1986; Ivancevich and Matteson, 1984).

Howard and his colleagues (1976) studied 300 top managers from 12 major Canadian companies to determine the prevalence of Type A behavior and risk factors for heart disease. Overall, 61 percent of the managers were classified as Type A's. The highest percentage of extreme Type A's were found in the 36–55 year age group. The Type A's had significantly higher serum lipids and blood pressure and more stress symptoms than the Type B's. In addition, more Type A's were cigarette smokers and less apt to exercise than Type B's.

Froggatt and Cotton (1987) did not find Type A individuals to be more likely than Type B individuals to feel stressed. Differences in stress between Type A and Type B occur because Type A individuals seek out situations that are objectively more stressful. Indeed, as Miles (1976) pointed out, the degree and type of role conflict a person experiences on the job is contingent upon the requirements of the role occupied. Role stressors appear to have detrimental health effects, but stressor effects are contingent on aspects of the person and the situation (Fusilier, Ganster, and Mayes, 1987). Not all individuals are equally vulnerable to the same potential stressors in the same work situation.

Benight and Kinicki (1988) studied the interaction between the personal characteristic of Type A behavior and the environmental factor of perceived controllability of stressors on two behavioral outcomes of stress: overt exhibition of Type A behavior and task performance. Subjects were divided into Type A/B categories and randomly assigned to either a moderately or highly uncontrollable managerial in-basket simulation. Results indicated that the personal characteristic of Type A behavior had its strongest effect on the overt exhibition of Type A behavior when subjects perceived their environment as moderately uncontrollable. Results also confirmed the prediction that environmental factors dominate personal characteristics in affecting stress outcomes when the situation is perceived as highly uncontrollable. As McLean (1979) has pointed out, both stressful events and stressful conditions exist within the work environment. In addition, there are stressful occupations, stress associated with the role of the person in an organization, stress associated with relationships at work, and stress associated with the organizational structure and climate at work. All of these sources of stress interact with the idiosyncracies of the individual personality to produce real or imagined stress. Burke and Deszca (1982) state that individuals are attracted to jobs and organizational climates which match their own stable behavioral and attitudinal properties.

Boundaries and boundary perceptions are an important part of work stress. Boundary role personnel in an organization serve both as filters and facilitators. They determine what information is processed and how their organization is represented externally. An organization relies upon the expertise and discretion of its boundary role personnel. They have a gatekeeper's power and may become even more powerful if the information they provide is vital to the organization's survival (Aldrich and Herker, 1977). Many studies emphasize the stress and conflict felt by personnel in boundary roles. There are also numerous sources of gratification to boundary spanning. Several studies have found very small or insignificant correlations between role conflict, role ambiguity, and boundary spanning activity. Aldrich and Herker (1977) argue that boundary spanning jobs enable boundary spanners to reduce uncertainties for others, to gain power, improve their bargaining position, increase their job satisfaction, and even gain better jobs.

Boundary Spanning and Personality

Table 4-1 lists possible personality characteristics and management styles and common management problems associated with managing different boundary situations. Managing flexible boundaries, or boundary spanning, is a middle range position between the extremes of rigidity and fluidity. For example, in surgical situations, the boundaries are quite rigid. Well-known protocols must be adhered to, and each member of the surgical team has specified roles. The personalities of surgical personnel are generally known to be controlling, directive, confrontational, aggressive and task-oriented. Most of us would not want our surgeons to be otherwise. At the other extreme, mental health personnel have to deal with a wide range of behaviors which often involve the unpredictability of clients. Therefore, they must be flexible, adaptive and, perhaps, indecisive until all facts are known. It is when the personality of the manager does not fit the situation and an inappropriate management style is used, that management problems ensue.

In any organizational setting, the leader is the one agent who has a significant impact on work activities. The work of McGregor and Argyris have emphasized the supportive aspects of leadership. These researchers have assumed that supportive leader behavior will increase performance and morale. Research work at Ohio State has indicated that both supportive and task-oriented leadership behaviors are needed to achieve personal organizational goals. The Ohio State leadership styles emphasize *consideration* (respect) and *initiating structure* (defining and structuring roles). Behling and Schriesheim (1976) found that supervisors giving more directions had lower-performing subordinates when they showed little consideration but higher performing subordinates when they showed a great deal of consideration.

TABLE 4-1

**Personality Characteristics and Management Styles of
Managers and Common Management Problems
Associated with Different Boundary Structures**

Boundary Structures

	Rigid Boundary	Flexible Boundary	Fluid Boundary
Personality Characteristics	Intolerant of ambiguity	Likes independence/ autonomy	Tolerant of ambiguity
	High internal locus of control	Flexibility	High external locus of control
	Type A personality	Good self-concept	Type B personality
	Need for control	Adaptable	Need to be liked by others
	Predictable behavior	Flexible	Impulsive behavior
	Confrontive	Arbitrative	Withdrawing
	Guarded/Protective	Openness	Ambivalence Indecisiveness
Management Styles	Directive	Compromising	Ameliorative
	Forceful	Participative/ Facilitative	Placating
Common Management Problems	High employee turn-over	Sufficient support from management	High employee turn-over
	Low morale	High morale	Low morale
	Little employee professional growth	Change requires negotiation of boundary adjustments	Little employee professional growth
	Boredom	Willingness of employees to change (to be flexible)	Employee job descriptions overlap
	Too little information flow inside/outside organization	Information exchange sufficient and effective	Too much information flow inside/ outside organization

Source: John G. Bruhn

It seems reasonable to assume that a leader's influence and how it is applied can be viewed as a stressor by individuals at different times. Leaders are also stressed by employee behaviors.

Table 4-1 is a list of possibilities which might be found along a boundary management continuum. It is likely that the personality facet of tolerance of ambiguity moderates stress. Individuals with a low tolerance for ambiguity who find themselves in a job or in organizational environments where there is little structure will be more likely to find that this situation generates role ambiguity and anxiety than would someone who tolerated ambiguity better. It appears that individuals who have a high need for structure, i.e., clearly spelled out boundaries, have less stress, are more satisfied, and perform their jobs better (Ivancevich and Mattson, 1980).

Like tolerance for ambiguity, locus of control may also seem to moderate stress. Locus of control refers to an individual's perception of the extent to which control over external stimuli resides within themselves or outside, beyond their influence. People who are internals perceive themselves as having more control over external events than people who are externals. Using role conflict as an example, the employee who is an internal will perceive that he or she has at least some control over that condition and will act to reduce its potency as a stressor. Externals, on the other hand, see no relationship between their behavior and control of the stressor.

There is reason to believe that locus of control is related to self-esteem. But managers who attempt to change an employee's locus of control or self-esteem will find them not easily changeable. The best approach toward providing a better match between the individual and the environment, is to reduce potential stressors, such as overly fluid or overly rigid boundaries.

Certainly, employers try to achieve good matches between the personalities of the workers they employ and the types of situations with which workers will have to deal. The more changeable a job situation, the more adaptable the employer and employees must be. Some types of jobs and professions that require a great deal of flexibility are marketing, personnel recruitment, labor relations, sales, finance, and purchasing. In the health professions, a distinction can be drawn between professionals who provide services only to patients and professionals who provide services to both patients and physicians. However, in the case of health professionals, such as pharmacists, physical therapists, occupational therapists, and nutritionists, who can serve patients directly as well as receive referrals from physicians, the boundaries of "ultimate responsibility" are not always clear.

Alaszewski (1977) refers to health professions which fall in between requiring a physician as manager and being independent contractors as "rootless specialties." All of the health specialties that deal with rehabilitation, for example, fall within this category. In Alaszewski's view, the intervention of "rootless specialists" creates a situation between medical patronage and paramedical independence. While both may co-exist, the degree of success in maintaining this boundary is highly dependent upon the personality and interpersonal skills of the specific health professional. Boundary spanning requires a high degree of tolerance of ambiguity and a tolerance for sharing power and control (leadership). These characteristics are essential for teams and make them successful or unsuccessful. Our current health problems are rarely sequestered within the neat boundaries of a specific health discipline. The problems of aging, AIDS, heart disease, cancer, and trauma all require boundary spanning if the patient's total treatment and rehabilitation are of the highest priority. Similarly, prevention and health education cannot be effectively and efficiently delegated to health educators alone. Boundary spanning activities in the health professions will increase in the future. Are we adequately educating future health professionals to be effective boundary spanners?

The Role of the Leader in Boundary Management

If all organizations essentially recapitulate the family structure, then leaders are psychologically in parent-like roles. The leader, as a surrogate parental figure in our culture, is significantly a teacher (Levinson, 1981). It is the task of leaders to define the purpose of the organization, to unite the purpose with the people who are involved, and to help employees pursue their own ego ideals. It is also the task of the leader to keep the organization current and dynamic so that it remains viable and competitive. The needs and roles of workers change as do the tasks that they perform. Just as a parent establishes and adjusts role boundaries within the changing family, the leader must guide and protect role boundaries in changing organizations.

Mergers, retirement, transfers, and promotion all disrupt role boundaries. Workers became angry and frustrated when their values are violated, when they have difficulty in coping with change, when they do not have a sense of forward movement, and when they cannot adequately work as they are used to. Leaders need to be careful managers of the egos of workers as boundaries change in an organization. Problems are compounded in an organization when there is inadequate information from the leadership and repetitive change in role boundaries. Helping workers maintain an equilibrium in their role boundaries in the face of change is a crucial and unavoidable task of leaders of modern organizations (Levinson, 1981).

Feijen (1990) discusses the social psychological paradox of the person who wants to distinguish himself and, at the same time, be one of the group. Distinguishing yourself means to take space for yourself, to do the things that fit you and that you like. Being one of the group means to subject yourself to the rules, standards, and values of the group to which you belong, but also to influence them. Boundary management involves maintaining the balance between rules and space.

Aldrich (1979) sees the need for organizations and their managers to change continually to perfect the fit between the organization and the environment in which it exists. Organizations must be responsive to the needs of the environment; therefore, organizational boundaries should not be so fixed that they cannot respond to change. As the proverb goes, "The tree which has grown up and become rigid is cut into lumber" (Heider, 1986, p. 151).

REFERENCES

Adorno, Theodor W., Frenkel-Brunswik, Else, Levinson, Daniel J. and Sanford, R. Nevitt: *The Authoritarian Personality.* New York, Harper, 1950.

Alaszewski, Andy: Doctors and paramedical workers—the changing pattern of interpersonal relations. *Health and Social Science Journal, 87:* B1–B4, October 14, 1977.

Aldrich, Howard: *Organizations and Environments.* Englewood Cliffs, Prentice-Hall, 1979.

Aldrich, Howard, and Herker, Diane: Boundary spanning roles and organizational structure. *Academy of Management Review, 2:* 217–230, 1977.

Argyris, Chris: *Overcoming Organizational Defenses: Facilitating Organizational Learning.* Boston, Allyn and Bacon, 1990.

Behling, Orlando, and Schreisheim, Chester: *Organizational Behavior: Theory, Research and Application.* Boston, Allyn and Bacon, 1976.

Benight, Charles C., and Kinicki, Angelo J.: Interaction of Type A behavior and perceived controllability of stressors on stress outcomes. *Journal of Vocational Behavior, 33:* 50–62, 1988.

Bennis, Warren, and Nanus, Burt: *Leaders: The Strategies for Taking Charge.* New York, Harper and Row, 1985.

Blake, Robert R., and Mouton, Jane S.: Reactions to intergroup competition under win-lose conditions. *Management Science, 7:* 420–435, 1961.

Blake, Robert R., and Mouton, Jane S.: *The Managerial Grid III.* Houston, Gulf Publishing, 1985.

Blake, Robert R., and Mouton, Jane S.: *Building a Dynamic Corporation through Grid Organization Development.* Reading, MA, Addison-Wesley, 1969.

Brown, Roger: *Social Psychology.* New York, Free Press, 1965.

Bruhn, John G.: Managerial indecisiveness: When the monkeys run the zoo. *Health Care Supervisor, 8:* 55–64, 1990.

Bruhn, John G.: Control, narcissism, and management style. *Health Care Supervisor, 9:* 43–52, 1991.

Bruhn, John G.: Administrators who cannot let go: The super manager syndrome. *Health Care Supervisor, 11:,* 1993.

Burger, Jerry M., McWard, Jennifer, and La Tolle, Dennis: Boundaries of self-control: Relinquishing control over aversive events. *Journal of Social and Clinical Psychology, 8:* 209–221, 1989.

Burke, Ronald J., and Deszca, Eugene: Preferred organizational climates of Type A individuals. *Journal of Vocational Behavior 21:* 50–59, 1982.

Caplan, Robert D., and Jones, Kenneth W.: Effects of work load, role ambiguity and personality Type A on anxiety, depression, and heart rate. *Journal of Applied Psychology, 60:* 713–719, 1975.

Dailey, Robert C.: Group, task, and personality correlates of boundary-spanning activities. *Human Relations, 32:* 273–285, 1979.

Feijen, René H. P. F.: Boundary management: A dynamic balance between rules and space. *Human Systems Management, 9:* 257–265, 1990.

Fiedler, Fred E.: *A Theory of Leadership Effectiveness.* New York, McGraw-Hill, 1967.

French, John R.P., and Caplan, Robert D.: Psychosocial factors in coronary heart disease. *Industrial Medicine, 39:* 383–397, 1970.

Frew, David R., and Bruning, Nealia S.: Perceived organizational characteristics and personality measures as predictors of stress/strain in the work place. *Journal of Management, 13:* 633–646, 1987.

Froggatt, Kirk L., and Cotton, John L.: The impact of Type A behavior pattern on role overload-induced stress and performance attributions. *Journal of Management, 13:* 87–98, 1987.

Fusilier, Marcelline R., Ganster, Daniel C., and Mayes, Bronston T.: Effects of social support, role stress, and locus of control on health. *Journal of Management, 13:* 517–528, 1987.

Garfield, Charles: *Peak Performers.* New York: Avon Books, 1986.

Gemmill, Gary, and Heisler, William: Machiavellianism as a factor in managerial job stain, job satisfaction, and upward mobility. *Academy of Management Journal, 15:* 51–64, 1972.

Gilmore, Thomas N.: Leadership and boundary management. *Journal of Applied Behavioral Science, 18:* 343–356, 1982.

Harrington, Kathryn R.: *Strategic Flexibility: A Management Guide for Strategic Times.* Lexington, D.C. Heath, 1985.

Harris, Jeffrey S., and Dewey, Mary Jane: Management of organizational stressors. In O'Donnell, Michael P. and Ainsworth, Thomas H. (eds.): *Health Promotion in the Workplace.* New York: Delmar, 1984.

Heider, John: *The Tao of Leadership.* Hampshire, England, Wildwood, 1986.

Hill, Percy H., Bedau, Hugo. A., Chechite, Richard A., Crochetiere, William J., Kellerman, Barbara L., Ounjian, Daniel, Pauker, Stephen G., Pauker, Susan P., and Rubin, Jeffrey Z. (eds.): *Making Decisions: A Multidisciplinary Introduction.* Reading, MA, Addison-Wesley, 1979.

Howard, John H., Cunningham, David A., and Rechnitzer, Peter A.: Health patterns associated with Type A behavior: A managerial population. *Journal of Human Stress, 2:* 24–31, 1976.

Howard, John H., Cunningham, David A., and Rechnitzer, Peter A.: Role ambiguity, Type A behavior, and job satisfaction: Moderating effects on cardiovascular and biochemical responses associated with coronary risk. *Journal of Applied Psychology 71:* 95–101, 1986.

Ivancevich, John M., and Matteson, Michael T.: *Stress and Work: A Managerial Perspective.* Glenview, IL, Scott, Foresman, 1980.

Ivancevich, John M., and Matteson, Michael T.: A Type A–B person-work environment interaction model for examining occupational stress and its consequences. *Human Relations, 37:* 491–513, 1984.

Jennings, E.E.: *An Anatomy of Leadership: Princes, Heroes and Supermen.* New York, Harper and Row, 1960.

Kast, Fremont E., and Rosenzweig, James E.: *Organization and Management: A Systems and Contingency Approach.* Fourth edition. New York: McGraw-Hill, 1985.

Kelly, Joe: *Organizational Behavior: Its Data, First Principles, and Applications.* Homewood, IL, Richard D. Irwin, 1980.

Kets De Vries, Manfred, F.R., and Miller, Danny: Personality, culture, and organization. *Academy of Management Review, 11:* 266–279, 1986.

Landau, Martin, and Stout, Russell: To manage is not to control: Or the folly of type II errors. *Public Administration Review, 39:* 148–156, 1979.

Levinson, Harry: Leadership and stress. In Meltzer, H., and Nord, Walter R. (eds.): *Making Organizations Humane and Productive: A Handbook for Practitioners.* New York, Wiley, 1981.

Maccoby, Michael: *The Gamesman.* New York, Simon and Schuster, 1976.

McLean, Alan: *Work Stress.* Reading, MA, Addison-Wesley, 1979.

Messing, Bob: *The Tao of Management.* Hampshire, England, Wildwood, 1989.

Miles, Robert G.: Role requirements as sources of organizational stress. *Journal of Applied Psychology, 61:* 172–179, 1976.

Miller, D., and Friesen, Peter H.: *Organizations: A Quantum View.* Englewood Cliffs, Prentice-Hall, 1984.

Miller, Danny, Kets De Vries, Manfred, F.R., and Toulouse, Jean-Marie: Top executive locus of control and its relationship to strategy-making, structure and environment. *Academy of Management Journal, 25:* 237–253, 1982.

Miller, Suzzane M.: Why having control reduces stress: If I can stop the roller coaster, I don't want to get off. In Garber, Judy, and Seligman, Martin E.P. (eds.): *Human Helplessness: Theory and Applications.* New York, Academic Press, 1980.

Oncken, William, and Wass, Donald L.: Management time: Who's got the monkey? *Harvard Business Review, 52:* 75–80, 1974.

Ouchi, William G.: *Theory Z.* New York, Avon Books, 1981.

Pascale, Richard Tanner: *Managing on the Edge.* New York, Simon and Schuster, 1990.

Phillips, Donald T.: *Lincoln on Leadership.* New York, Warner Books, 1992.

Pierpaoli, Paul G.: Management diplomacy: Myths and methods. *American Journal of Hospital Pharmacy, 44:* 297–304, 1987.

Schein, Edgar H.: *Organizational Psychology.* Engelwood Cliffs, Prentice-Hall, 1972.

Seligman, Martin E.P.: *Helplessness: On Depression, Development and Death.* San Francisco, Freeman, 1975.

Sheldon, Alan: *Organizational Issues in Health Care Management.* New York: Spectrum, 1975.

Siegel, Jacob: Machiavellianism: M.B.A.'s and managers: Leadership correlates and socialization effects. *Academy of Management Journal, 16:* 404–412, 1973.

Spotts, James V.: The problem of leadership: A look at some recent findings of behavioral science research. In Eddy, William B., Burke, W. Warner, Dupre, Vladimir A., and South, Oron P. (eds.): *Behavioral Science and the Manager's Role.* Washington, DC, NTL Institute for Applied Behavioral Sciences, 1969.

Tannenbaum, Robert, and Schmidt, Warren H.: How to choose a leadership pattern. *Harvard Business Review, 51:* 162–180, 1973.

Volkart, Edmund H. (ed.): *Social Behavior and Personality.* New York, Social Science Research Council, 1951.

Chapter 5

BOUNDARY CONFLICTS IN ORGANIZATIONS AND GROUPS

An individual's conscious or subconscious definition of his
own boundaries may play an important part in his success—
or lack of it.

Nancy Foy (1980)
The Yin and Yang of Organizations

Disputes within and between organizations can usually be traced to concerns related to boundary control. Individuals and organizations carefully guard boundaries, which they believe define their jobs or missions, against intrusions and change. Miller and Rice (1973) have clearly stated the issue:

> Without adequate boundary definitions for activity systems and groups, organizational boundaries are difficult to define and frontier skirmishing is inevitable . . . the more boundaries can be located, the more easily communication systems can be established. Unless a boundary is adequately located, different people will draw it in different places and, hence, there will be confusion between inside and outside. In the individual, this confusion leads to breakdown; in enterprises, to inefficiency and failure (p. 42).

Boundary skirmishes occur, even when boundaries are clearly defined, because social change continually modifies boundaries. When change occurs, needs change, requiring assessment of the new needs and of how they can be met. This often requires the rearrangement of boundaries.

Boundary perception and boundary control are intimately tied to the needs of individuals. Needs for power, control and recognition influence the effectiveness with which individuals protect their boundaries and the extent to which they seek out opportunities to expand their boundaries. The thoroughness with which boundaries are protected determines whether organizations function effectively or, indeed, survive. The aggressiveness with which boundaries are expanded determines whether organizations grow or maintain their status quo.

Health institutions and health professionals experience a great deal of change. Boundaries continually are threatened. Competition for patient and research dollars and rising health care costs create the need to challenge and change deeply entrenched and carefully controlled boundaries. Increased specialization, shortages of certain types of health personnel, and the creation of new specialties have resulted in boundary changes within the health professions. Societal demands for equal opportunity, accessibility, and affordability continually challenge the boundaries of the entire health enterprise, demanding a more open system. These demands and changes have had a measurable impact on the management and effectiveness of all health organizations, from small hospitals to large health science centers.

Types of Boundaries

Boundaries in organizations can be characterized in many different ways. Schein (1971) has identified three types of boundaries that characterize the internal structure of an organization: 1) hierarchical boundaries, which separate levels from one another; 2) inclusion boundaries, which separate individuals or groups who differ in their degree of centrality; and 3) functional or departmental boundaries, which separate departments, divisions, or other groups from one another.

Boundaries can vary in number, degree of permeability, and type of filtering properties. For example, in the military, functional boundaries separate different line and staff activities, but rotating officers to keep them highly flexible have made these boundaries permeable; people move from function to function. On the other hand, a hospital's functional boundaries, which correspond to different clinical departments, are impermeable; a physical therapist would not be moved to a Department of Ophthalmology. While a small business or private practice may have very few functional boundaries, these are very permeable because one or two people perform all the functions.

Hierarchical or inclusion boundaries, which separate levels in organizations, vary in permeability. For example, the proliferation of new technologies and techniques, such as the artificial kidney, high voltage x-ray therapy, and ultrasound, have led to increased specialization in the health care field. New occupations have developed—for example, ultrasound technicians and nuclear magnetic imaging technologists. The desire to gain increased recognition and income have led the personnel in these new fields to seek validation through certification and licensure.

Other inclusion and functional boundaries are delineated by: continuing education requirements, peer review, codes of ethics, grievance committees, professional standards review organizations, and periodic recertification. Yet, as Gross (1984) notes, such policies may be self-serving; professionals charged with regulating themselves to protect the public evoke the image of a fox guarding a hen house.

The mechanisms that influence entry into systems, both for clients and professionals, are a source of boundaries and a reinforcer of boundaries. The problem of *entry* is fundamental and pervasive in individual and organizational life. For the individual, the problem is one of *getting in*, gaining admission to school or to a professional society. Getting a job means achieving entry into a work organization (Schein, 1971). A service organization's entry system determines the character and composition of the client population that will receive services. For instance, to obtain the services of a mental health organization, initially, one must go through an "intake" procedure in which applicants are screened and selectively admitted. Rejected applicants may or may not receive a referral to another source of care (Levinson and Astrachan, 1991).

One function of the entry system is the regulation of patient input. Some clinical facilities, whether or not they offer appropriate services, are legally required to accept for treatment every applicant who meets certain eligibility requirements. In such cases, admission units cannot adequately control their boundaries. When admissions are too generous, boundaries can be protected by neglecting, transferring, or discharging unwelcome patients early. Admission units may "overcontrol" boundaries, admitting only a special group of applicants. Private hospitals, seeking to limit costs associated with uninsured or inadequately insured patients, may limit admissions or seek to transfer patients. The residency "culture" in public hospitals may discourage admissions to control the "work load." On the other hand, a person who has insurance may be admitted to the hospital even though the needed treatments could be given at home.

As Levinson and Astrachan (1991) point out, the entry system should be more than a sieve or gatekeeper. Persons seeking health care cross various boundaries. Their entry experiences can help to shape, positively or negatively, their subsequent experiences as patients. If the admission process is to be more humane, greater attention must be given to admission as an organizational problem.

Boundaries within hierarchies, and functional groups in organizations, can be conceptualized according to their changeability. Not only can boundaries be impermeable or permeable, they can change or become nonexistent. All of us are familiar with organizations that maintain strict, impermeable boundaries (e.g., seminaries, the military, parochial schools, libraries, and hospitals) and situations that require the maintenance of rigid boundaries (e.g., surgery, church services). Leaders in organizations with boundaries that are inflexible and cannot be crossed maintain a high degree of control over members; innovation and creativity are discouraged and the status quo becomes tradition.

Organizations and institutions that are known for their impermeability have difficulty adapting to change. When medical schools were pressured by outside groups to admit more ethnic minorities, some administrators and faculty members resisted (and still resist), claiming that many minority students did not meet competitive standards for admission, especially with respect to grades and admission test scores. They were reluctant to consider any criteria other than the quantitative. The medical college admission test (MCAT) has not shown a strong correlation with clinical performance in medical school, but has continued, as a matter of tradition, to be used as an admission requirement. Admission to most health professions programs still is carefully controlled.

Organizations and institutions that have permeable boundaries are the most common. This doesn't mean that no rule controls the behavior of members, rather that exceptions to the rule are tolerated and considered. Students who encounter a crisis and miss an exam can be permitted to make it up, a conscientious employee who has used all his/her sick leave and has a medical emergency can be retained on the payroll, or an employee can make up time taken from work for a personal appointment. These are examples of accommodations to the rules that control boundaries. It is the manager's responsibility to oversee boundaries so that they are neither too rigid nor too fluid. In either extreme, employees can become frustrated and leave the organization.

When situations, rather than pre-established rules, determine boundaries, employees continually test boundary limits as new situations arise. This leads to poor morale among employees who compare their treatment by management in given situations with the experiences of fellow employees. Managers who want to be liked by all employees often are the culprits in boundary mismanagement of this type.

Preferential treatment in a store where people are waited on in an order other than that in which they arrive is a common example of what can happen when boundaries are fluid. Patrons angered by such treatment probably will disavow any loyalty to that store. In hospital emergency rooms, the triage method is used to determine which patients will be seen first. Yet, patients with insurance, or those known by one of the staff, may be seen rapidly regardless of their complaints. Patients who irritate the staff by complaining, or who suffer from a complaint considered trivial by the staff, will be put at the end of the line.

Organizations with no boundaries do not exist for long. An organization that lacks basic structure will die by its own actions or inaction. For example, organizations sprang up in many cities as a result of the growing AIDS crisis and, with the best of intentions, some took on too many activities and burned out. Others were unable to focus on a constructive way to help handle the crisis, but seemed obsessed with anger and frustration resulting from societal reactions to AIDS. Members joined and left such organizations, forming new ones based upon their personal concerns. As a result, organizations with a common purpose competed or fought with each other over scarce financial resources or problems of common concern. Another example might be that of a political campaign that failed because its organizers had no clearly established boundaries: workers shared no plans, the only thing they had in common was their liking for a specific candidate.

While organizations need focus to give them shape and coherence, too narrow a focus will result in their failure to use the talents of their members and their loss of potential recruits. On a personal level, eliminating some rigid boundaries can open up new options. Wilber (1981) claims that new discoveries and personal growth occur only after people become dissatisfied with their life boundaries and develop a "no-boundary awareness," which permits them to see things in a new way.

Boundaries Between Organizations

Freeman (1978) notes that changes in organizations, both over time and through space, complicate the problem of defining organizational boundaries. Over time, organizations grow, merge with other organizations, acquire subsidiaries, or change goals and identities. Organizations either can be independent units or members of large organizational systems.

Whether an organization is freestanding or part of a multiorganizational system may influence its use of boundary-spanning strategies. Fennell and Alexander (1987) used data from a national survey, conducted, in

1982, by the American Hospital Association, to study the boundary-spanning strategies of freestanding hospitals and members of multi-organizational hospital systems. Of 1,411 acute care, community hospitals, 901 responded. Hospitals in systems were more likely to bridge boundaries, probably because corporate policies were designed to centralize functions and minimize costs. Bridging between members of multihospital systems is easier than bridging by individual hospitals to other hospitals outside hospital systems. The researchers also found that hospitals appear to have a higher propensity to join a multihospital system in states where the model is strong, and that the hospital system is highly fragmented: hospitals have no uniform, predictable response to external pressures, different segments of the industry are influenced by different types of pressure. However, increased regulatory stringency did not contribute to system joining on the part of a hospital. Regulatory programs do not appear to be a way to "push" hospitals toward greater reliance on other organizations. Membership in a multihospital system is not a protective measure against regulatory pressure. Hospitals tend to respond to external regulatory pressures by developing complex boundary strategies, such as retrenchment at the administrative rather than the technical care level. Protection of technical care may also explain why hospitals in regulated environments are less likely to join multihospital systems, and why clinical services are less likely than other hospital services to develop bridges to other organizations. Both of these strategies involve restructuring technical care. Hospitals, when faced with outside pressures, are more willing to sacrifice layers of administrative buffering than to relinquish control of clinical services.

Hospitals, typically, are closed systems. Most hospital managers tend to be "boundary fighters" who protect their territory and, because they fear that change will diminish their power and prestige, defend the status quo. Boundary fights occur when leadership is unable to structure boundaries around the institution's mission and protect its core from dilution or erosion. Therefore, hospital managers tend to be conservative, sometimes rigid, and resistant to change.

Boundaries must be strong enough to maintain responsible behavior within an organization, but permeable enough to allow cooperation between discrete organizations working toward a common goal. Boundaries are "real" in the sense that they influence behavior. For example, some typists are afraid to correct their supervisors' awkward sentences because they believe they have no "right" to change their supervisors' words, while others compose their supervisors' correspondence from hastily written notes. The difference in their behavior results from the different ways in which their supervisors have defined the boundaries of their job responsibilities. Although boundaries may be artificial human creations, it is necessary that they be clarified and understood; otherwise conflicts ensue. By "standing at the boundary," a manager creates a controllable world, a world in which activities are relatively predictable and organized and can, therefore, be coordinated to respond to an uncertain and changing world.

The stability of an organization's boundary is determined largely by the boundary manager, in this case, the hospital's CEO. When management is unable or unwilling to set boundaries, individuals within the organization attempt to redefine/define, clarify/reclarify the organization's mission in order to contain personal anxieties. This "reinterpretation" often leads to the creation of individual tasks that oppose the organizational mission. For example, although a hospital may originally have been founded as an indigent care facility, financial constraints may lead to policies that effectively exclude charity patients.

Boundaries that are not clearly defined, and are frequently changed, result in confusion. For example, most intensive care units are managed by specially trained nurses, who are much more knowledgeable than the primary care residents who rotate through the units. Supposedly, the nurses are to request guidance from the residents when supervising physicians are not available. However, it is generally understood that the "suggestions" nurses make to residents are more than just suggestions. The residents, especially first year residents, are in the ICU's to learn. Some residents do not understand the boundaries of their roles. Unless the physician director of the ICU makes the boundaries of resident decision-making clear, patient care may suffer. Individual employees, in extreme cases, may have so many conflicting perceptions of boundary limits that they render an organization ineffective. On the other hand, the boundary limits of an organization may be drawn so severely that the organization becomes disconnected from related organizations, resulting in poor communication, lost and poorly served consumers, and open, fierce competition for essential resources.

The management of organizational boundaries effectively calls upon three major traits: 1) the ability to maintain a strong organizational culture; 2) the ability to anticipate the need for, and lead the way toward, change; and 3) the ability to manage ambiguity. Peters and Waterman

(1982) observed that well-managed companies have strong cultures, the consequence of having leaders who, for many years, hammer away at particular sets of cultural beliefs in messages to their organization. A strong organizational culture emphasizes a reciprocal relationship between leaders and followers in their mutual task of meeting organizational objectives; both "give" and both "receive" something from this coalition (Bass, 1985).

Kanter (1983) calls those managers and organizations who are adept at the art of anticipating the need for, and leading the way to, productive change, change masters. Innovating organizations have ambiguities, overlaps, decision conflicts, and decision vacuums in some parts of the organization. Some uncertainties, however, create opportunities. Kanter notes that innovative organizations have a culture of pride characterized by open communication, utilized networks, and decentralized resources. A culture of pride creates a propensity for risk-taking, which, in turn, produces more innovation and a self-reinforcing cycle. Kanter states, "life is not perfect in innovating organizations, but at least the tools exist for individuals to use to make corrective changes." An effective manager must manage the paradoxical condition of ambiguity; too much ambiguity creates confusion and uncertainty, too little creates a feeling of entrapment and inability to grow. Ambiguity exists in an organization when the information (role definition and feedback) is inadequate to do a job properly. Since the threshold of ambiguity differs for each individual employee and manager, an organization's CEO must continually monitor the ambiguity tolerance level of the organization and periodically redefine or restructure it. Rumors among the employees of impending changes in the organization are a common indication that the limits of ambiguity need to be redefined. Changes in leadership create an especially difficult time for an organization. Boundaries shift; decisions, such as hiring, that used to be reserved for top management, may be shifted downward. Decisions, such as adherence to safety regulations, that once were made at the middle management level, may be shifted upward. Increased periods of organizational anxiety occur when the environment for organizational functioning changes greatly. Health professions facilities and educational institutions face periods of uncertainty when legislation alters funding sources and sets new requirements for educational programs.

Foy (1980) notes, the job of a manager is to shift the boundaries, both inside and out, to make sure others can work effectively, anticipating boundary problems and diverting them. The manager also needs to be an amplifier for the employees, translating and promoting their ideas to the world outside their boundaries.

Conflict-Prone and Conflict-Resistant Organizations

Stokols (1992) studied the ways in which various facets of group and organizational structure promote, prevent, or moderate the intensity and health consequences of interpersonal conflict. He noted that few interpersonal conflicts occur in a socially or organizationally neutral context. Stokols hypothesized that physical environmental arrangements and social conditions within some organizations predispose their members toward chronic conflict and health problems, whereas the qualities of other organizations make interpersonal conflict less likely. Conflict-prone and conflict-resistant organizations have three distinguishing characteristics: 1) the social-psychological qualities of groups, which include norms, common goals, and members' expectations about their roles and the roles of others; 2) the organizational structure, which includes interrelations among members' roles and the processes by which they are managed; and 3) environmental conditions external to the group that exert a stabilizing or destabilizing influence on the organization's social structure and internal processes. Social-psychological qualities of organizations that may predispose their members to conflict include the absence of shared goals, incompatibilities between individuals' personal styles and role assignments, and rigid ideologies. Boulding (1972) emphasizes the importance of cohesion, the need to maintain a consistent structure of roles that can be filled with reasonably satisfied persons, especially as an organization grows. An organization with rewarding roles will be stable internally. Boulding also notes that an organization's self-image, the value it places on expansion and competition, relates to potential conflict in the organization. Organizations frequently organize themselves against something. A strong enemy can be a unifying force for an organization, wherein employees feel participation in a larger purpose.

Compatibilities among group members' styles of work and their tasks encourage cooperation rather than hostility. Blake and Mouton (1984) note that membership pride, group loyalty, and a group's investment in its own success help to create a conflict-resistant organization. Kahn (1972) indicates that an organization is made up of an array of overlapping role sets. Conflicts can arise in response to excessive overlap between tasks and uncertainty about the way work is evaluated. According to Kahn, the issue is not to eliminate conflict and ambiguity from an organization, but to contain it.

The availability and arrangement of physical resources within organizations also can predispose a group to conflict or cooperation. Invidious comparisons between groups, regarding space, personnel, resources, attributed motivations, and hearsay, can cause people to act on their assumptions about one another. A win-lose philosophy in an organization can help to heighten these comparisons. Blake and Mouton (1984) suggest a variety of ways to resolve interface differences between groups in organizations. These include cooperation, by managerial edict, in negotiation, personnel rotation, leadership replacement, structural changes, establishing liaisons, mediation and arbitration, flexible reporting relationships, and bringing in an outsider to act as an interpersonal facilitator. As Blake and Mouton note, these interventions help to promote communication in an organization, and communication permits us to get at causes, not in communication, but in the *values* embraced by the organization and its employees.

Odiorne (1981) indicates that an organization's leader often attempts to seek an egalitarian approach to conflict. Management may attempt to seek concurrence about an issue to maintain morale, rather than improve decision-making in the organization. This concurrence-seeking, referred to as "groupthink," occurs when a cohesive "in group" seeks to retain its unity and overrides any dissident opinion or suggestion of alternatives.

Another distinguishing characteristic of the conflict-resistant organization is its large number of "good soldiers." Organ (1988) has characterized organizational citizenship behavior as discretionary, not directly or explicitly recognized by the formal reward system, and promotive of the effective functioning of the organization. While the creation of "good soldiers" is labeled altruistic by some, a strong organizational culture, a participatory climate whereby supervisors and employees share common goals and ideas, and a reward system that invests in people, contributes to a unique conscientiousness that employees feel and share.

Boundary Change and Boundary Fighting

Boundaries do not always remain fixed, they change by design or are modified by events. How boundaries are maintained and the degree to which they change directly relates to the personal needs of the person who manages them. The less the boundary manager's personal need to control, the more likely boundaries are to change.

Social and technological change can also change the boundaries within an organization. Crises or catastrophes can cause organizations to reorganize and rethink previous boundaries. Since boundaries are perceptions, boundaries change because as people change, so do their perceptions. As people and circumstances change, a program, project, policy, or organization may be abolished because it no longer meets a need. For example, difficult financial times may cause a community to consider merging competing organizations that have similar goals, e.g., Boy's Club and Y.M.C.A.

People change boundaries, and boundaries change people's behavior. Boundaries become issues when people perceive them to be threatened or attacked by boundary fighters from within or without an organization. Organizations with permeable, fluid, or nonexistent boundaries are easy prey for boundary fighters. How well a boundary is managed influences how easily a boundary can be transgressed. While people aggressively try to intrude on new boundary territory, their major reason is a desire to broaden their scope of power and control (Bruhn, 1991; Bruhn and Lewis, 1992). Broadening one's sphere of control indicates success and elicits recognition.

Situations Conducive to Boundary Fighting

Boundary fighting exists in health organizations and institutions, just as it does in the non-health world, and can affect, directly, the quality of service and consumer satisfaction. Table 5-1 lists some common situations that help bring about boundary fighting.

Change (or stagnation) in organizations, and leaders who are perceived to be weak encourage boundary fighting. These situations are not unique to hospitals and other health care organizations. Since most health care and educational institutions are closed systems, and it is important for the managers of closed systems to maintain stability in their organizations, it is essential to control external threats to that stability. The "public image" of hospitals and health science centers is conservative and their "public language," for the most part, dissuades boundary fighters from the outside. New methods for delivering health care have occurred through the emergence of new institutions, e.g., Health Maintenance Organizations.

Changes in the education of health professionals have been minimal

TABLE 5-1
Situations Conducive to Boundary Fighting

▼ Leadership transitions in a unit, department, organization or institution

▼ An administrative unit is not meeting the needs and priorities of an organization and/ or its employees

▼ Weak leadership (personality and style) and poorly defined boundaries

▼ Individual achievement is rewarded over teamwork and cooperation

▼ Low employee morale, high turn-over rate

▼ Frequent changes of leadership

▼ Frequent changes in the mission, priorities, structure, or operational methods of an organization

▼ The personal needs of a leader for power, control, and recognition

▼ The lack of decision-making by leaders

▼ Changes in operating procedures (new policies, reclassification of titles and pay scales, etc.) without input from the rank and file.

▼ The withdrawal of support for leaders by employees and their displacement of anger and frustration on undoing the organization through passive-aggressive behavior, gossip, etc.

▼ Opportunity for professional growth of personnel or growth of the organization or group is limited

▼ Scapegoating and unwillingness of administrators to take responsibility for weaknesses and potential problems

▼ Persons having too many jobs or roles in an organization

Source: John G. Bruhn

and carefully controlled by the agencies that accredit health professions education programs. Tradition still pervades all of health care, services, and education. Despite growing public debate and concern about the three "A's" of health—accessibility, availability, and affordability—politically powerful professional organizations, through their lobbyists, have dissuaded most individuals who wish to modify boundaries. Attempts to modify boundaries within health organizations and institutions is carefully managed to "keep things under control." This controlled work or study climate discourages innovation and creativity, especially if workers challenge established procedures or methods. Particularly discouraged are those actions that appear to question the authority, power, or control of organizational leaders.

Most boundary management focuses on 'putting out fires' in boundary skirmishes among health care workers, professionals, students, and administrators. Perhaps the best example of a common skirmish is the one generated by the crisis created, in some hospitals, by the shortage of nurses, necessitating the closure of hospital beds and operating rooms. The recruitment of nurses to the U.S. from other countries and the consideration of a new type of nurse (registered care technician) by the American Medical Association have created boundary conflicts among nurses as well as between nurses and physicians (Homolka, 1990; Cherwenka, 1990). The leaders of hospitals and nursing programs have made the assumption that the missions and tasks of nurses and physicians are clearly defined; however, the missions and tasks of each group include protecting the sanctity of its boundaries.

There are numerous examples of "turf" disputes between health professionals, e.g., occupational therapists and physiatrists, psychiatrists and psychologists, nurse anesthetists and anesthesiologists, anesthesiologists and surgeons, medical technologists and pathologists, occupational therapists and physical therapists, nurse practitioners and physician's assistants, etc. Most of these disputes result from discrepancies in compensation between disciplines which perform similar tasks and from different degrees of autonomy between related disciplines. Many of the boundary issues between the noted disciplines have existed for years, and while they differ in intensity, from place to place, health administrators are aware of potential skirmishes and must maintain "administrative buffer" zones to prevent destructive skirmishes.

Boundary disputes can consume the majority of a manager's time, leaving little time for planning or creative thinking. As Blanchard,

Oncken and Burrows (1989) said, . . . "there are always more monkeys clamoring for attention than we have time to manage, unless we are extremely careful about which ones we accept responsibility for, it is very easy to wind up caring for the wrong monkeys while the really important ones are starving for lack of attention" (p.130). Boundary management in an organization, including the management of boundaries between managers, is perhaps the most time-consuming activity of an administrator.

Gilmore (1990) has written that leadership is different from management. Leadership requires using power to influence the thoughts and actions of other people. Leadership involves creating conditions in which people can work effectively and from which poachers will be discouraged. The manager, on the other hand, is a problem solver. Managers and leaders differ in their world views. The dimensions for assessing these differences include their orientation toward their goals, their work, their human relations, and themselves (Zaleznik, 1977). Clear boundaries must be drawn to reduce uncertainty and anxiety about what is expected of employees. Change is an aspect of life; it is a leader's responsibility to anticipate and plan for change in the spaces and overlaps between tasks so that boundaries do not become problems. As Gilmore (1990) said, "it is like trying to ride a bicycle and build it at the same time" (p.137). Too often, in health care settings, we focus on managing, rather than on providing leadership that is willing to clearly delineate boundaries and expectations. We focus on building the bicycle and rarely experience what it is like to ride it.

Symptoms of Boundary Fighting

Boundary fighting creates feelings of anxiety, which can lead to anger and aggression. One function of boundaries is the containment of anxiety. Established rules and procedures provide structure for work, and give employees some degree of security and sameness. Boundaries provide standards, which help employees assess their accomplishments and determine whether they are fulfilling management's expectations. When boundaries are threatened or changed, the status quo is disturbed, routines are disrupted, and uncertainty about the future is created, resulting in varying degrees of anxiety. Employees may become defensive, cliquish, and begin to gossip, speculate, and project their feelings onto others. Communication becomes indirect and employees spend a great deal of time sharing their fears. Some employees cope with their anxiety by withdrawing from others, determined to ensure their job security by increasing their involvement in their work.

Persistent anxiety may erupt in the form of anger, especially if an employee believes that there has been a direct intrusion into his/her territory. Some employees may test boundaries to see how far they can go and become labeled as "troublemakers." Angry responses from fellow employees are usually a sign that one has intruded into sensitive territory. Aggressive reactions are often the end result.

Physical space is an important boundary marker, indicating power and prestige. The need for more space indicates the growth of an organizational unit, and growth, in most organizations, is a laudable objective. Acquiring more space is, therefore, a direct or indirect objective of most managers. Medical schools, for example, recruit new department chairs with promises of more space, more faculty, and more equipment. Anchor or key departments are "given" space, while other, smaller departments have to "fight for" space. Those who have more space also have more resources and, as a result, acquire even more space. Less "prestigious" areas, which do not bring many financial resources to an institution, are usually given less desirable space. Perhaps the most frequent instances of boundary fighting occur when space is shared by two or more departments or divisions, each of which regards the space as theirs.

Boundary Conflicts Among Health Disciplines in the Hospital

Extraordinary advances in radiology have allowed radiologic services to transcend their traditional role to one that involves both diagnosis and treatment. This has given rise to major issues of "turf."

Clinicians and non-physicians have become involved in forming and owning imaging centers, formulating their policies, and performing imaging procedures. As regulations sought to limit the distribution of these technologic advances in institutions, physicians sought to ensure their ability to perform these procedures, own and/or control this instrumentation, and interpret and receive proper compensation for their efforts (James et al., 1990). Therefore, radiologists have had to respond to continuing challenges of "turf."

Challenges to turf in ultrasonography, especially in obstetrics and gynecology, cardiac ultrasonography, and more recently, carotid flow studies involving neurologic sciences, have evolved into significant conflicts. As a result, ultrasonographic services have been underused, even when instrumentation was available. Improper use of ultrasonographic equipment has resulted from a lack of knowledge or inadequate training, and overuse has resulted from self-referral.

Magnetic resonance imaging (MRI) has caused renewed analysis of issues regarding antitrust, the regulation of distribution of and access to technological equipment, and considerations of competence, standards of care, and turf among specialties, especially in academic institutions (James et al., 1990). MRI's clinical introduction and growth took place in an economic climate which continued to place emphasis on free enterprise and entrepreneurship. Initially, favorable tax laws, economic incentives, and a plentiful supply of investment money favored the formation of joint ventures and limited partnerships, both in academic and private settings. The complex relationships of ownership and patient care provide ground for new antitrust considerations and issues of turf.

Another phenomenon that leads to turf considerations is that of exclusive contracts. Antitrust legislation primarily was enacted to prevent the abuse of market power (turf). Medicine has at least two markets, one geographical and the other product-related, and academic settings have a third, teaching resources. Market power may be exercised by a single, dominant or by a collective contracting group; for example, a hospital and a radiology group with an exclusive contract to provide a defined service could exercise market control.

Numerous measures must be considered when formulating an exclusive contract. Separating technical and professional fee schedules, refusing to engage in contributions to the parent institution, and identifying the existence of termination agreements between the contracting parties are important boundary issues.

Another turf battle has emerged regarding the motivations for self-referral. Many physicians have incorporated imaging technologies into their office practices. Diagnostic-related groups' (DRG) method of reimbursing hospitals for inpatient stays resulted in the expansion of outpatient services, including imaging technology. The potential harm to radiologists of the increasing frequency of self-referral by non-radiologist physicians is evident (Hillman, 1991). Proponents of self-referral argue that performing imaging in their own facilities is quicker and easier for the patient. The counter argument is that self-referral is likely to result in poorer quality imaging, less expertise in interpretation, and ethical conflicts for physicians who have a financial incentive to refer patients to their own facilities. To illustrate the complexity of boundary interfaces between radiologists and non-radiologist physicians, Levin and Matteucci (1990) report:

> A survey of nonacademic community hospitals was conducted to ascertain the degree of control radiologists have of 38 selected imaging or imaging-related interventional procedures. Responses from 187 hospitals showed that community hospital radiologists totally controlled or strongly dominated almost half of these procedures, including all computed tomographic and magnetic imaging studies, bone radiography, breast needle localization, emergency department radiography, arthrography, obstetric ultrasound, renal and peripheral angroplasty, percutaneous abscess and biliary drainage, percutaneous nephrostomy, cerebral angiography, and interventional, neuroangiography . . . from more than the 500 procedure codes used by radiologists, 38 were chosen as representing potential areas for "turf battles" (p.321 and 324).

Discussions of turf involve perceived rights. In a rapidly evolving and expanding discipline like radiology, it is difficult to establish legal standards for professional competence and quality control. Technology, when it opens the door for new ways to control human disease, also opens the door for opportunistic gatekeepers of health care to increase their status, power, prestige, and economic position.

Boundary Conflicts in Academic Health Centers

Rogers (1978) discusses numerous problems encountered by academic medical centers, among them the medicalization of social problems. He notes that many problems, in the last decade, which seem to have emerged in response to the stresses, strains, and shortfalls of modern society, have been moved into the preview of medicine. These include overuse of alcohol, addiction to drugs, violence, child abuse, sexual identity problems, marital incomparability, behavioral disorders, compulsive overeating, and even gambling. In the past, these were viewed as moral problems, and individuals suffering from them were viewed as morally corrupt. However, the moral values approach makes it extremely difficult to agree upon solutions. Furthermore, the judgment of moral corruption makes it difficult for the individuals involved to seek change and rehabilitation. Viewing these social problems as medical problems permits people to shift the blame from themselves to society, or to a constitutional weakness, and to view themselves as victims, like people suffering from a common infection, rather than as active collaborators in their illness. Many problems are trivialized by using an illness metaphor.

The medical metaphor tends to diminish the power of personal choice. While the medical metaphor may improve the prospect of rehabilitation for those subject to these problems, it might excuse the development of such "moral problems" in individuals who, in a more censorious day, would successfully resist the impulses that lead to problem behavior. Many problems encompass more than the personal weaknesses that can be conceptualized as fitting the medical model. Unhappy home life, unemployment, poverty, social alienation, and stress play a role in their origins. Some medical schools have established new departments of sociomedical science or social medicine to handle them. The complex nature of these problems, and their roots outside the classic concepts of disease, mean they cannot be solved within the medical model. They have been moved to medicine by default because the medical center seems to be the only game in town (Rogers, 1978).

Because the increase in these problems has accompanied the development of late 20th century society, the medical profession is under pressure to expand its boundaries to include areas of mental and spiritual health that have been avoided by medicine since the development of modern science. The outcome of these pressures on the medical profession and medical education is still unknown.

The problems these ailments create for the academic medical center are enormous. Affected individuals represent a high percentage of those who attend ambulatory clinics and emergency rooms. External forces, in Rogers' view, have helped reshape and expand the boundaries of health science centers. Rogers proposes cooperative linkages between health science centers, government, hospitals, and the private sector and an end to adversarial positions. He suggests that academic health science centers must adopt missions that are broader than some centers might wish, yet narrower than society demands of them.

Akin to the complex boundary interfaces between health science centers and other institutions, are the boundaries that exist between departments or units within the academic health center. Figure 5-1 shows the various boundary interfaces between schools and faculties collaborating to offer a Master of Public Health degree in one Australian university. The degree is made possible by the cooperation of two schools in the Faculty of Medicine (School of Community Medicine and School of Medical Education) and the School of Health Sciences Management in the Faculty of Professional Studies in teaching courses and advising students. Students also can take courses on an elective basis in the Graduate School of Management, which is not part of the Faculty of Medicine. While this program demonstrates that several parties can cross boundaries to cooperate in facilitating a course of study, it also points out fragile interdependencies that exist between the academic units offering the degree. The quality of the degree is entirely dependent upon the quality of boundary crossing in teaching and advising.

Another type of boundary crossing is common in academic health science centers. Figure 5-2 shows hypothetical relationships between four areas of focus in an academic health science center: professional service, research, teaching, and clinical practice. A contemporary faculty member who expects to be promoted and tenured should spend time in all four areas. Professional services is perhaps the most amenable of the four areas of focus to boundary crossing. The shared abilities and skills required by professional services tend to be generic rather than attributable to specific disciplines. Research can be a collaborative effort, depending on the problem. However, most research efforts, in academic health science centers, especially in the basic sciences, remain competitive within disciplines. The most difficult area in which to cross boundaries is that of clinical practice; subspecializations, which exist within disciplines, severely restrict clinical practice's susceptibility to boundary crossing. Teaching, on the other hand, offers the opportunity to tackle problems that involve several disciplines, e.g., cancer, coronary heart disease. Team teaching is now common within and between disciplines. Didactic teaching, in contrast to the one-on-one teaching that takes place in clinical practice, can involve several techniques and occur in a variety of settings.

Figure 5-2 shows why it is more difficult to work in some of the four areas of focus than others. It is necessary that people feel secure in the knowledge and skills relating to their own discipline before they can comfortably cross boundaries in teaching, research, and professional service. It might be hypothesized that clinicians, who seek out interdisciplinary situations and group practices, are the most aggressive and successful of boundary crossers.

FIGURE 5-1

Boundary Interfaces in Offering a Degree with Several "Homes"

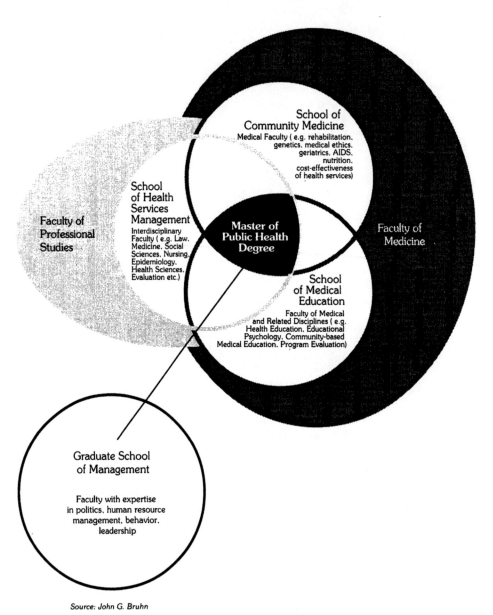

Source: John G. Bruhn

FIGURE 5-2

Hypothetical Representation of Degrees of Difficulty in Crossing Boundaries in Academic Health Science Centers

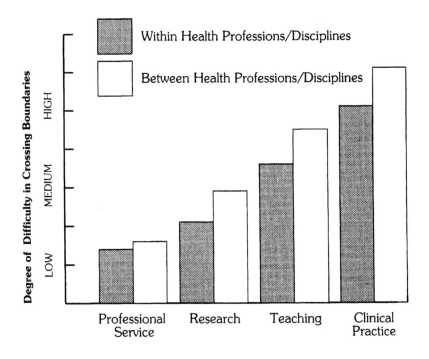

Areas of Faculty Concern in Academic Health Science Centers

Source: John G. Bruhn

Non-traditional Jobs and Boundary Crossing

Two phenomena are apparent when individuals move into occupations previously associated with members of the opposite sex. The first derives from gender and division of labor, differentiation by function, and subsequently by occupation. This differentiation creates boundaries around particular kinds of work that limit entry into that work to members of one sex. Individuals are assigned to these occupations according to sex, and members of the same culture generally share beliefs about who belongs in that occupation. The second facet of the phenomenon derives from structure, position, and status. This facet also reflects shared norms within a culture, but it pertains to the *value* attached to a particular occupation. In our culture, occupations and tasks traditionally assigned to men usually acquire and carry more value or prestige than those assigned to women (Schreiber, 1979).

Gender typing of jobs is a matter of established fact. Its negative impact on career opportunities for women has received extensive attention, but men also face limiting factors due to the societal and personal barriers that discriminate against free vocational choice. According to reports, men in nursing, child care, and early childhood education encounter strong prejudice (Chusmir, 1990). Societal disapproval and sex-related discrimination on the job are accepted facts. Yet, more men are choosing to enter female-dominated occupations. Chusmir (1990) found that women who choose careers in male-dominated occupations are likely to possess many of the personality and motivational traits commonly attributed to men. A parallel pattern was found for men who choose careers in female-dominated occupations.

Adaptations and adjustments may be made by organizations and individuals to deal with the potential problems of gender incongruity. It is not unusual, for example, for women in male-dominated careers to specialize in acceptable functions within the normally male occupation. Female lawyers often choose family law, female doctors specialize in obstetrics and gynecology and pediatrics, and female dentists commonly practice on children. In the same way, personnel directors and career counselors suggest that men in nursing who are concerned with problems of gender incongruity concentrate their efforts in anesthesiology, urology, or radiology.

Much of the research in nontraditional career choice has focused on its impact on individuals. However, organizations are also affected by this type of boundary crossing. For example, Schreiber (1980) found that males were more readily accepted into female work groups than vice versa; there was greater resistance to females coming into male work groups. This finding has direct implications for group morale, productivity and job satisfaction.

Motivations for Boundary Conflict

Every decision we make, every action we take, every word we speak is based, consciously or unconsciously, on the construction of boundaries. Boundaries exist only when we construct them. Boundaries establish opposites. To draw boundaries is to manufacture opposites (Wilber, 1981). The world of opposites is a world of conflict. Every boundary line is also a battle line. The firmer the boundaries, the deeper the conflicts. We consistently try to alter boundaries to remove their constricting power.

Boundaries are a product of our perceptions. We regard our perceptions as real and accurate and act on them. Therefore, the boundaries we perceive are real. We frequently assume that life would improve if certain boundaries were eliminated.

Boundaries are seen as impediments to power and status. People cannot increase their power and status without the opportunity for upward mobility or movement. Boundaries, perceived or real, prevent mobility, heighten frustration and dissatisfaction, and lead individuals, groups, and organizations to take overt action to create new opportunities for advancement. This involves confronting boundaries that are perceived to be impediments to power and status.

Studies have found, for example, that hospitals with effective reward systems are more likely to retain nurses than hospitals without effective reward systems (Bennis, Berkowitz, and Malone, 1958). Sandefur (1981) noted that the higher the level of organization-specific resources, the more likely an individual is to move upward within organizational boundaries. When an organization does not provide clear-cut channels for advancement, highly motivated personnel search for other employment opportunities.

The current shortage of nurses provides an example of boundary challenging. Hospitals overtly challenge each other's boundaries to recruit nurses, offering large sign-on bonuses and other fringe benefits. While this open-warfare may help to solve the acute shortages of nurses, it does not help health care personnel foster organizational loyalty, nor does it solve the basic problems underlying the nursing shortage. It might be argued that, while a nursing shortage exists, nurses benefit monetarily, but monetary rewards are a diversion from the real basis for power and status among the health professions. The shortage of hospital nurses has caused hospital CEO's, especially in hospitals which are state supported, to up the ante to compete with private hospitals for personnel. Many private hospitals have large numbers of vacant beds due to increased costs of operation. Fewer patients can afford the cost of care. Thus, either new alliances or open warfare are created among hospitals as they compete for patients.

People strive for positively valued social identity, e.g., they aspire to membership in groups that compare favorably with other groups. Ellemers and her colleagues (1988) found that members of high status groups showed more in-group identification than members of low status groups. Members of low status groups with permeable boundaries identified less with their group members than did members of low status groups with impermeable boundaries. The desire to enhance one's status is most strongly expressed when ingroup identification is decreased and upward mobility is a real prospect.

These findings apply to the various allied health disciplines, in a medical setting, that have low status compared to that of physicians, but have varying status among themselves, e.g., a physical therapist has higher status than a physical therapy assistant, and a physical therapy assistant has higher status than a recreational therapist. Higher status among disciplines is achieved by increasing entry requirements for admission to the field, maintaining strong control over accreditation requirements for educating personnel, and maintaining strict control over the number of schools and the size of classes, ensuring that shortages exist and salaries in the field remain inflated.

Boundary conflicts occur when marked pay differentials exist among allied health personnel with similar qualifications who perform related functions in the same setting, e.g., occupational therapists and physical therapists, nurse practitioners and physician's assistants. Groups tighten their boundaries to retain their power and status and to prevent less qualified personnel, even within their own discipline, from entering the ranks with minimal effort, e.g., physical therapy assistants becoming physical therapists. As boundaries in the health professions are drawn more tightly, opportunities for interdisciplinary collaboration lessen and the chances for conflict increase.

Kanter and Stein (1979) have noted that people build investments in organizations that may have little to do with the organization's goal. As individuals, groups, and organizations focus on enhancing their power and status by crossing boundaries, they become more concerned with rewards than with the primary reasons for their existence. One general guideline for preventing boundary conflicts is to ensure that an organization and its members not lose sight of their purpose and periodically renew themselves.

REFERENCES

Bass, Bernard M.: *Leadership and Performance Beyond Expectations.* New York, Free Press, 1985.

Bennis, Warren G., Berkowitz, Norman, Affinito, Mona and Malone, Mary: Authority, power, and ability to influence. *Human Relations, 11:* 143–155, 1958.

Blake, Robert R. and Mouton, Jane S.: *Solving Costly Organizational Conflicts.* San Francisco, Jossey-Bass, 1984.

Blanchard, Kenneth, Oncken, William Jr., and Burrows, Hal: *The One Minute Manager Meets the Monkey.* New York, William Morrow, 1989.

Boulding Kenneth E.: The organization as a party to conflict. In Thomas, John M. and Bennis, Warren G. (Eds.): *Management of Change and Conflict.* Baltimore, Penguin, 1972.

Bruhn, John G.: Control, narcissism, and management style. *Health Care Supervisor, 9:* 43–52, 1991.

Bruhn, John G. and Lewis, Raymond: Boundary fighting: Territorial conflicts in health organizations. *Health Care Supervisor, 10:* 56–65, 1992.

Cherwenka, Doris I.: Nurses oppose registered care technician recruitment. *Journal of the American Medical Association, 263:* 1860, 1990.

Chusmir, Leonard H.: Men who make nontraditional career choices. *Journal of Counseling and Development, 69:* 11–16, 1990.

Ellemers, Naomi, van Knippenberg, Ad, de Vires, Nanne and Wilke, Henk: Social identification and permeability of group boundaries. *European Journal of Social Psychology, 18:* 497–513, 1988.

Fennell, Mary L. and Alexander, Jefferey A.: Organizational boundary spanning in institutionalized environments. *Academy of Management Journal, 30:* 456–476, 1987.

Foy, Nancy: *The Yin and Yang of Organizations.* New York, William Morrow, 1980.

Freeman, John H.: The unit of analysis in organizational research. In Meyer, Marshall W. (Ed.): *Environments and Organizations.* San Francisco, Jossey-Bass, 1978.

Gilmore, Thomas N.: Effective leadership during organizational transitions. *Nursing Economics, 8:* 135–141, 1990.

Gross, Stanley J.: *Of Foxes and Hen Houses: Licensing and the Health Professions.* Westport, Quorum, 1984.

Hillman, Bruce J. Whose turf is imaging? Independent practice, academics, and research. *American Journal of Roentgenology, 156:* 443–447, 1991.

Homolka, Chuck: Registered care technicians can ease nurses' tasks. *Journal of the American Medical Association, 263:* 1861, 1990.

James, A. Everett, Curran, William J., Pendergrass, Henry P. and Chapman, John E.: Academic radiology, turf conflict and antitrust laws. *Investigative Radiology, 25:* 200–202, 1990.

Kahn, Robert L.: The management of organizational stress. In Thomas, John M. and Bennis, Warren G. (Eds.): *Management of Change and Conflict.* Baltimore, Penguin, 1972.

Kanter, Rosabeth Moss and Stein, Barry A. (Eds.): *Life in Organizations: Workplaces as People Experience Them.* New York, Basic Books, 1979.

Kanter, Rosabeth Moss: *The Change Masters.* New York, Simon and Schuster, 1983.

Levin, David C. and Matteucci, Theresa: "Turf battles" over imaging and interventional procedures in community hospitals: Survey results. *Radiology, 176:* 321–324, 1990.

Levinson, Daniel L. and Astrachan, Boris M.: Organizational boundaries: Entry into the mental health center. *Administration and Policy in Mental Health, 18:* 433–446, 1991.

Miller, Eric J., and Rice, A. Kenneth: *Systems of Organizations: The Control of Task and Sentient Boundaries.* London, Tavistock Publications, 1973.

Odiorne, George S.: *The Change Resisters.* Englewood Cliffs, Prentice-Hall, 1981.

Organ, Dennis: *Organizational Citizenship Behavior: The Good Soldier Syndrome.* Lexington, D.C. Heath, 1988.

Peters, Thomas J. and Waterman, Robert H. Jr.: *In Search of Excellence.* New York, Warner, 1982.

Rogers, David E.: *American Medicine: Challenge for the 1980's.* Cambridge, Ballinger, 1978.

Sandefur, Gary D.: Organizational boundaries and upward job shifts. *Social Science Research, 10:* 67–82, 1981.

Schein, Edgar H.: Organizational socialization and the profession of management. *Industrial Management Review, 9:* 1–15, 1968.

Schein, Edgar H.: The individual, the organization, and the career: A conceptual scheme. *Journal of Applied Behavioral Science, 7:* 401–426, 1971.

Schreiber, Carol Tropp: *Changing Places: Men and Women in Transitional Occupations.* Cambridge, MIT Press, 1979.

Stokols, Daniel: Conflict-prone and conflict-resistant organizations. In Friedman, Howard S. (Ed.): *Hostility, Coping and Health.* Washington, American Psychological Association, 1992.

Wilber, Ken: *No Boundary.* Boston, MA: New Science Library, 1981.

Zaleznik, Abraham: Managers and leaders: Are they different? *Harvard Business Review, 55:* 67–78, 1977.

Chapter 6

EFFECTS OF ORGANIZATIONAL
CHANGE ON BOUNDARY MANAGEMENT

> In the end change begets change. Technology, economy,
> and government stimulate organizational response, and
> that response pummels an organization into new and unex-
> pected shapes.
>
> *Carol Tropp Schreiber*
> Changing Places

Organizations, like individuals, avoid change. Kanter (1989) has said,
"The traditional large, hierarchical corporation is not innovative
or responsive enough; it becomes set in its ways, riddled with pecking-
order politics, and closed to new ideas or outside influences ... " When
change does occur, most people are pleased with the changes they,
themselves, have brought about because they adapt as they change
(Odiorne, 1981). The more change can be controlled, the less disruptive
it is. One reason change is resisted, and is disruptive when it does occur,
is the fact that boundaries change.

Change implies giving up something to which a person is committed
and which he/she values (Schein, 1969). Change is resisted because
change implies that existing behaviors and attitudes are wrong or
inadequate. Change that is imposed is usually more disruptive than
change that is planned by those whom it affects. Schein (1969) has
described a three step process of change that involves unlearning, or
unfreezing, cognitive redefinition, and refreezing. Just as unfreezing is
necessary to begin change, refreezing is necessary for change to endure.

Perhaps one of the most difficult changes an organization can make is
to alter its structure and mission. Such changes are disruptive because
they change how people work and how they perceive the value of their
work. Hospitals are an example of organizations that are currently undergoing structural and mission changes.

Reshaping Organizational Mission and Structure

Urban Public Hospitals

Urban public hospitals are significant providers of primary care and ambulatory care, and are responsible for training a significant proportion of our country's health care professionals. After 1950, the vitality of many urban public hospitals began to decline. The population served by the hospitals increasingly became poorer and more dependent. The departure of the middle class from inner cities eroded their tax bases, and local governments could no longer afford to support public hospitals at their previous levels. During the 1950's, urban public hospitals lost leading medical research staff and faculty. The demand for hospital services changed.

In the 1980's, many long-standing problems of urban hospitals worsened, and new ones surfaced. The undercapitalization of public hospitals remains a significant difficulty. Cutbacks in Medicaid eligibility, coupled with severe unemployment and an influx of immigrants, led to an increase in the number of uninsured urban residents. Reports of "dumping" these uninsured patients, transferring them from private to public hospitals, have become frequent (Altman *et al.,* 1989).

The role and scope of urban public hospitals have changed and so have their boundaries. Most of their problems have been imposed by social, economic and governmental change. Urban public hospitals have attempted to retain their identities and enhance their survival through mergers, joint ventures, consolidated service functions, reformed payment plans, and aggressive marketing strategies. Altman and his colleagues (1989) studied four public hospitals in four different geographic areas of the United States in an attempt to understand what policy variables influenced their performance. They concluded that there is no quick fix for the problems faced by urban public hospitals. Since urban public hospitals remain attached to their local political structures, the most important factors influencing their financial structures, as well as the quality of care they provide, are the fiscal condition of their state and local governments and the attitude of their communities toward the public hospital system. Changes in reimbursement policies have a disproportionate effect on public hospital systems. The boundaries of the public hospital currently are fragile and tentative.

For-Profit Hospitals

The differences between for-profit and not-for-profit hospitals are becoming harder and harder to discern. The for-profit hospitals, being independent, are setting the pace of change. Corporate hospital chains steadily are expanding their share of the total hospital inventory. By 1991, one in four nonfederal acute care hospitals was investor-owned (Lindorff, 1992). With current vacancy rates at many hospitals as high as 50 percent, it is likely that more chains will become subsidiaries of larger firms. They will continue to push medical care in the direction of centralized ownership and management.

Boundaries within and between hospitals and health care professionals are changing markedly. Because of cost control policies, health professionals have less control over patient care. Institutional goals and financial policies and operations now are largely removed from local control. Decisions on the resource needs of physicians practicing in hospitals are not made simply on the basis of medical need, financial considerations dominate. As corporate chains build hospitals, they use their own criteria for determining who is competent. Hospital companies recognize that if they want to control costs, they must gain the upper hand in determining how, and how much, care is delivered to patients, and which patients will be treated. Choosing which doctors will practice at a hospital increasingly is determined by corporate chains through hospital medical committees on which management sit (Lindorff, 1992).

Doctors are being used as "gatekeepers" or "boundary managers" for insurance plans, which offer physicians bonuses for minimizing referrals to specialists and for minimizing hospitalizations. Doctors who practice at chain hospitals are required to accept the terms of insurance plans, which may include lower fee schedules than those of other insurers. As the number of physicians continues to grow, and the hospital industry gains in its control of patient flow, doctors who resist efforts at control will face competition with a hospital (Lindorff, 1992).

Academic Medical Centers

Rogers (1978) notes that many academic medical centers in the U.S. are situated in the middle of inner city slums. These hospitals, which historically treated the sick poor, have since expanded their mission beyond providing care and teaching to include research. There has been an exodus of patients and health professionals from the inner city to the suburbs. Hospitals have been overwhelmed by uninsured inner city patients who cannot afford hospitalization and use the emergency room as an alternative to outpatient clinics for ambulatory care.

As Rogers points out, academic medical centers did not create these problems; however, they have been slow to adapt to the needs of the inner cities and the increasing dependence of their population on the academic medical center for care. The boundaries of the inner city and society have moved inward at academic medical centers to an uninterested audience. Rogers (1978) states:

> To ask a physician or a trained hospital executive to do this kind of task (improve the climate or locale so that the inner city population can function more effectively) does not make sense. They need to pilot the important and demanding affairs of science, teaching, and patient care. Clearly, these institutions must have a "Mr. Inside." But perhaps a "Mr. Outside" should now play a more prominent role in meshing the institution more closely with its community and society (p. 93).

While Rogers acknowledges that some leaders of academic medical centers are now addressing themselves to the problems of the quality of life outside as well as inside their institutions' walls, the boundaries of the academic medical center have been guarded with fortress-like zeal as the gap between the sick poor and the providers of health care continues to widen.

Lewis and Sheps (1983) state that today our health care system is a loose structure of diverse interest groups and power centers without systematic relationships. Power is divided and shared among a wide range of private and governmental bodies. Each has some influence in deciding how the system functions. Some power centers are strong; others are weak. Not all groups are interested in all issues, but each tries to preserve its own power and thus tends to resist change. Major policy decisions are usually reached by bargaining and forming alliances in which not all participants are of equal strength. The health care system is riddled with conflicts over boundaries between those who provide health services and those who need health services.

Wilson and McLaughlin (1984) point out that paradoxes, complexity, ambiguity, and conflict are common descriptors of the academic health science center. The dean of the medical school is a boundary person. Much of the dean's mental energy is concentrated on addressing issues regarding the boundary between the organization and its external environment (see Figure 6-1). The dean must represent the institution to its public, its sponsors, its supporters, and its detractors. In addition, the dean must be a planner, a strategist, a bonding person, and a linking person, all of which are related to the role of a problem-solver (Wilson and McLaughlin, 1984). Thus, the dean is a pacesetter for change as well as the key person who monitors its direction and speed.

It is clear that the system of governance of the academic medical center is not working well. Wilson *et al.* 1980 made the following statement:

> Medical school deans often find themselves in this dilemma: people outside the institution push for intraorganizational change, and simultaneously there are pressures from the inside to maintain the status quo and insulate the organization from external influences. In addition, public policy tends to reflect an oversimplified *ad seriatim* view of problems: insufficient directed or applied research, a shortage of physicians in some areas, and quotas for primary care physicians are examples of such perceptions (p. 105).

The present organization and governance of the typical academic medical center is not properly adapted to solving the issues that face it at all levels. As Lewis and Sheps (1983) have said, "the health care crisis is not a crisis of knowledge, facilities, health personnel, or money. It is a crisis of organization, a crisis of planning, a crisis of relationships" (p. 1). "If it is to carry out its social obligations effectively, the academic medical center must cease to be a loose federation of duchies and principalities" (p. 214).

Residency Education

Boundaries also are changing for clinical education. There is concern that the current distribution of health professionals does not match national needs, and that the medical educational system is not responsive to the changing health care environment (Anderson *et al.*, 1989). This is especially true of residency education. We may be training too many specialists and too few physicians in certain areas, such as geriatrics. There also is concern that clinical education is not responsive to evolving patterns in health care delivery. Students are not being trained in settings, such as health maintenance organizations and free standing ambulatory clinics, where the demand for services is increasing. Because there is no centralized method for controlling graduate education programs, any change in content in education programs is likely to be piecemeal and disjointed. Anderson and his colleagues (1989) propose four steps for financing clinical education: 1) eliminate third-party payments for all costs associated with clinical education training programs;

FIGURE 6-1

Internal and External Demands on a Medical School

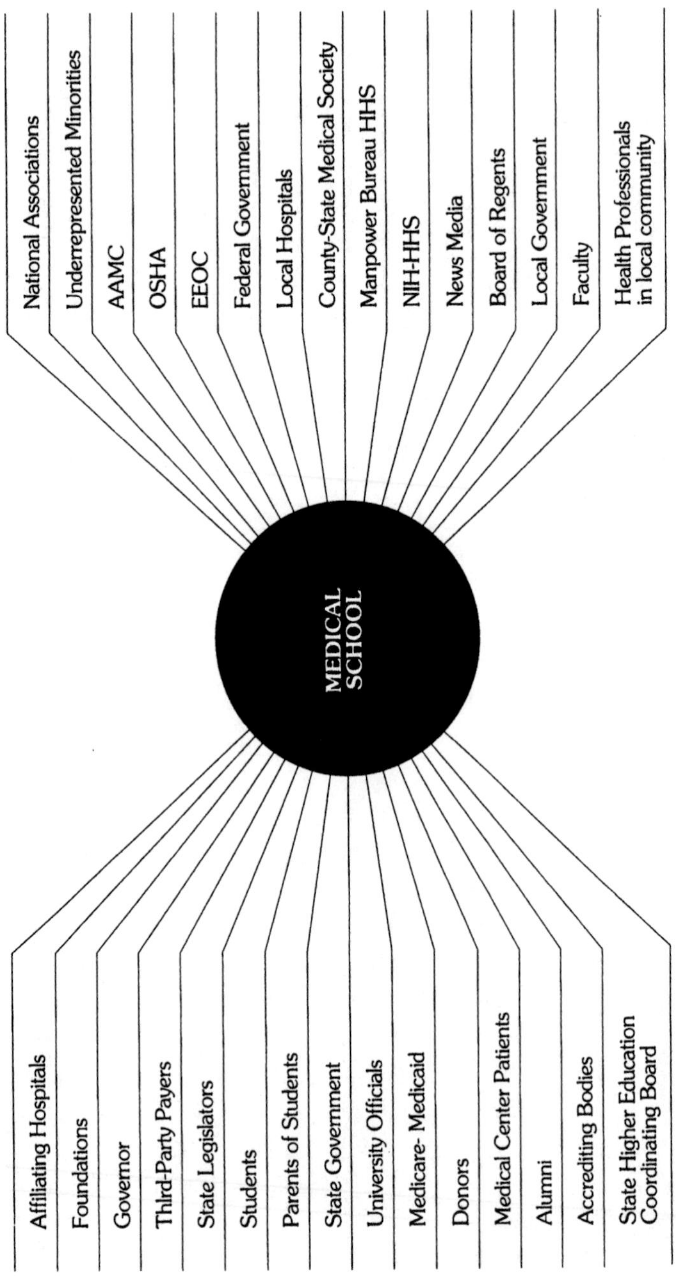

National Associations
Underrepresented Minorities
AAMC
OSHA
EEOC
Federal Government
Local Hospitals
County-State Medical Society
Manpower Bureau HHS
NIH-HHS
News Media
Board of Regents
Local Government
Faculty
Health Professionals in local community

MEDICAL SCHOOL

Affiliating Hospitals
Foundations
Governor
Third-Party Payers
State Legislators
Students
Parents of Students
State Government
University Officials
Medicare- Medicaid
Donors
Medical Center Patients
Alumni
Accrediting Bodies
State Higher Education Coordinating Board

*Modified from Wilson. Marjorie Price and McLaughlin,Curtis P.. *Leadership and Management in Academic Medicine*. San Francisco, CA.: Jossey-Bass. 1984. p. 29.

2) allow all personal and identifiable services performed by residents in an accredited program to be billed on a fee-for-service basis; 3) establish specific requirements for the supervision of residents; and 4) government intervention is needed to fulfill specialty and geographic requirements. Each of these suggestions has marked implications for existing boundaries between medical schools and the government.

Residency education supports many inappropriate and outdated boundary divisions and conflicts. Internal medicine, family medicine, and pediatrics all train generalists with little collaboration or discussion. For example, adolescent patients usually are treated by family physicians who receive little training in the developmental issues so important in assessing adolescents. Mentally ill or disturbed patients visit generalists before they consult psychiatrists, but psychiatric training for generalists is weak. Relationships between surgeons and generalists often are strained, but few attempts to resolve their conflicts have been made.

Ordinarily, decisions about the content of curricula in residency programs are made solely by the subspecialists involved, with limited output from other groups. Such "tunnel vision" does little to improve the care of patients, which is the raison d'etre for medical education. The ultimate solution to these problems might require more aggressive activities by groups, such as the American Board of Medical Specialties and the Society of Adolescent Medicine, which have a stake in collaboration among specialties.

Clinical Specialties

According to Coile (1990), the war of competition among hospitals and physicians will be fought in the "techno-niches" of clinical specialties. The market focus will increasingly use technology for market advantage. The market will focus on specialized high-tech facilities that the average community hospital will use to compete in a crowded marketplace. Every hospital over 200 beds will feature at least one specialty.

Recruiting medical superstars, for specialty niches, is a shortcut to market dominance. In 1987, Good Samaritan Medical Center of Los Angeles recruited Southern California's top cardiac surgeon from St. Vincent's. In one year, 400 open-heart surgical procedures were swung to Good Samaritan, and St. Vincent's, which previously housed California's busiest cardiac program, lost 33% of its revenue. Good Samaritan's revenues soared 15% in 1988 (Coile, 1990).

Techno-niche programs that feature high-tech procedures, such as laser surgery, have today's highest profit potential. The changing demographics of the U.S. population help drive niche markets. For example, the elderly, whose numbers are growing, demand services in rehabilitation, urology, oncology, and lithotripsy.

Problem-Oriented Learning in Medical Schools

Several medical schools have altered the structure and content of their curricula, shifting from a factual to a problem-based orientation. The movement to substitute problem-based learning for the traditional lecture systems in medical schools arises partly in response to the boundaries between basic and clinical scientists in teaching medicine. In order to encourage research, the teaching loads of basic scientists often consist of a few lectures during the year. Basic scientists often talk about their research interests with little concern about how to relate their lectures to the actual learning needs of medical students (Stemmler, 1989).

As a result, medical students are apathetic, even hostile, to basic science and to research careers. The late 20th century is one of the greatest scientific eras in human history, with the work in molecular biology providing astonishing new insights into the baffling phenomena of human pathophysiology. Yet, most medical students seem to regard basic science as the domain of a strange group of humans addicted to peering through microscopes, who are uneasy with human contact, speak an undecipherable jargon understood only by their research companions, and work in domains unlikely to have any important applications to the practice of medicine.

The present classes of medical students are unlikely to practice medicine tomorrow with the insights and tools of today. Changes in the amount of new information and the tools of information processing are proceeding to alter almost all professions, destroying great companies and creating new ones, changing the normal human life span, and altering human relationships worldwide. Medical information has to change as well, to increase the students' appreciation of science, their abilities to handle new knowledge, and their desire to grow and change with new discoveries.

Problem-based learning (PBL), which integrates basic science and clinical subjects, is organized around problems rather than disciplines, emphasizing the interpersonal and humanistic aspects of the practice of medicine in addition to cognitive skills. One assumption underlying

PBL is that once one has become a successful problem-solver one can tackle and solve a variety of problems (Norman, 1988). This assumption is somewhat problematic, but PBL's have been shown to increase student interest and motivation and the students' recall of solutions to various medical problems (Norman and Schmidt, 1992). Problem-based learning can be introduced into an established school or into a conventional curriculum, but several medical schools have chosen to redesign their entire curriculum, for example, Sherbrook Medical School in Quebec, which changed its entire medical school to problem-based learning in one year (Walton and Matthews, 1989). McMaster University, in Ontario, was a pioneer in PBL and restructured its medical curriculum in the early 1970's.

Problem-based learning raises many boundary issues among disciplines, which usually compete for time in the curriculum as well as space, faculty, and other resources. Perhaps a key issue in introducing problem-based learning in a medical school is convincing faculty members to give up the role of "the expert in control" in order for learning to take place. Some medical schools have introduced separate problem-based learning tracks, thereby avoiding having to move the entire teaching staff and student body to a PBL curriculum at one time, and providing a way to "test" faculty and student receptivity to PBL. U.S. medical schools that have implemented PBL include the University of New Mexico, Michigan State University, Rush Medical College, and Bowman Gray.

Faculty who "teach" in a PBL curriculum must reconstruct many boundaries, those vis-a-vis their colleagues in the same discipline, especially if all do not teach in the PBL curriculum, as well as with colleagues in other disciplines, who become more like team members. Since PBL, at least initially, takes a large commitment of faculty time, faculty will have less time to conduct research and publish, which means the institution will have to alter guidelines for promotion and tenure. Students also must alter their expectations of faculty, who become mentors and resource persons rather than "spoon feeders." Student-faculty interaction becomes more collegial, and trusting. Students can learn in a variety of ways, which provides greater flexibility in teaching and learning.

Szasz (1969) describes a project at the University of British Columbia's Health Sciences Centre in which an interdisciplinary committee, composed of faculty from medicine, nursing, dentistry, pharmacy, rehabilitation, social work, psychology, and home economics, planned a series of education experiments to increase awareness of the need for a comprehensive approach to a broad spectrum of human problems (interprofessionalization). They experimented with lectures offered to combined classes of students from various professions; learning experiences were offered in the framework of seminars, rounds, conferences, projects, field work, which utilized a variety of techniques including role playing and videotapes. Evaluation was difficult, but after two years Szasz and his colleagues (1969) tentatively concluded:

- Utilizing the problem-solving method in learning experiences appears to be the most promising means of developing collaborative relationships.
- Students of one profession react positively to students of other professions in their classes if the need to have common learning experiences is explained; conversely, they tend to resent or ignore students of another discipline or group if the reason for their presence is not made clear.
- In classes that contain representatives of more than one profession, without specially arranged opportunities for interaction, students do not discuss their educational experiences with students from other professions and, in fact, do not talk to each other on any topics.

We learn professional and disciplinary boundaries early in our education; these are reinforced by the learning environment, teaching techniques, and role models to which we are exposed. To achieve changes in boundary behavior in the classroom or in practice, it is necessary to restructure our organizations and institutions to convey the need to work together to solve common problems and, indeed, to plan how to prevent problems of common concern.

Management by Committees

Affirmative Action/Equal Opportunity

Affirmative action originally began as a series of presidential directives designed to encourage the recruitment of qualified minorities and women through advertising and training programs. Title VII of the Civil Rights Act of 1964 extended protection against discrimination in employment on the basis of an individual's race, color, religion, sex, or national origin. Under the old version of affirmative action, women and minorities attracted to an applicant pool would compete on a nondiscriminatory, colorblind, gender-neutral basis for jobs, promotions, or educational positions (Lynch, 1989). However, the goal of equal opportunity has been progressively abandoned in favor of a new, more radical version of affirmative action that emphasizes equality of results. Women and minorities are hired in proportion to their numbers in labor pools in the general population.

Proponents of the new, proportionally based affirmative action have tried to avoid the term "quotas." Quotas have not been viewed favorably by the courts. Therefore, almost every affirmative action plan refers to goals and timetables. However, in organizational practice, goals and timetables have often become quotas, used to rapidly boost the percentage of women or minorities and exclude better qualified Whites, especially White males (Lynch, 1989).

In 1985, Nathan Glazer reexamined the status of affirmative action. He endorsed the policy of preferential affirmative action for a limited time, but stressed the need to correct the education problems which have presented substantial barriers to occupational and economic development, especially for Blacks. By 1988, Glazer noted that affirmative action had been institutionalized in business and government.

While affirmative action has been successful in achieving greater racial and gender equity in the workforce, boundaries are clearer for ethnicity than for gender. For example, a university may set aside a few faculty positions specifically to encourage the hiring of ethnic minority faculty. Therefore, the need for ethnic diversity is explicitly advertised. On the other hand, women and handicapped applicants may be encouraged to apply for positions, but none are specifically reserved for them. These distinctions have caused some feelings of resentment even among underrepresented groups. The boundaries of affirmative action need to be carefully monitored by the EEO officer and institutional affirmative action committee in each setting. The EEO officer is the boundary manager between underrepresented groups and their employer.

In the 1977, U.S. Department of Labor 4th edition of the *Dictionary of Occupational Titles,* all references to sex and age in job titles and descriptions were eliminated, e.g., clergyman became clergy, newsboys became newspaper carriers, airline stewardesses became flight attendants. There are an increasing number of women in the labor force and some women occupy positions previously held mainly by men, e.g., bartenders, airline pilots. On the other hand, men are being hired for positions previously held mainly by women, e.g., telephone operators, librarians.

Schreiber (1979) studied a large company in the northeastern U.S. to assess the effects of a labor force in which men and women could change places. She found that the social situation rather than personality or gender was the major influence in how employees were treated in the organization. However, there was one significant, sex-linked difference related to expectations about promotion, women had lower expectations regarding future promotions than men working in the same job.

Role strain theory suggests that discrepancy between gender identity or sexual self-identification and occupational stereotyping should result in defensiveness and anxiety. Empirical evidence, however, does not confirm these expectations. Kadushin (1976) surveyed 259 male social workers and reported that they did not find their status to be troublesome. Choosing a non-traditional, gender-atypical career involves the interaction of numerous factors, personal, family, and societal influences. Successfully crossing occupational boundaries appears to be a function of the interaction of people's adaptive repertoire and style in specific social situations, which occur in the specific organizations where they are employed. Obviously, the philosophy and attitude of the management of an organization will set the stage for the receptivity of employees who cross occupational boundaries.

Today's emphasis on the culture of the workplace alerts us to the unstated and unobserved impediments to women's ability to work at the highest capacity and to have confidence in their capabilities (Epstein, 1970). Cultures prescribe attitudes and styles of behavior that become fixed as norms defining social roles. Norms also prescribe the kinds of behavior appropriate to gender roles. Epstein (1981) points out that most women are competitive, but she found, when interviewing female lawyers, that they rarely admit this and do not believe their sex is competitive. Women hold stereotyped views about themselves that damage their confidence.

There are social and psychological reasons for this behavior. Individuals do not want to stand out as deviants from their groups' norms; punishments for doing so range from eye raising to ostracism. Punishments can be ongoing, as people are reminded that they are non-conformists. Most contemporary cultures generally send messages that women are not as capable as men, irrespective of contrary evidence. The resources of institutions also affect receptivity to women. When resources are generous, women meet with more opportunity and good will. Although gender boundaries are changing, Zuckerman (1991) states, " . . . differences in early socialization and in the structure of opportunity (as reflected in the differential reward structure) have produced differences in expectations about work . . . even so recent evidence suggests that the gap . . . is narrowing:" (p. 70).

Other changes in the workforce are altering the boundaries of the past. Ethnic diversity is growing, more people with disabilities are employed, an increasing gap exists between highly educated persons and the large number of persons who cannot read and write well enough to hold simple jobs, and employees' values are becoming more personal and divergent (Jamieson and O'Mara, 1991). The realities and beliefs of the past, based on years of experience with a predominantly homogeneous workforce, shaped management's mindset.

Creating a new workplace will require planned organizational change. There is a need to design more responsive workplaces that will train managers and employees to value diversity, to individualize performance management, to align rewards with employees' values, to share information and encourage participation, to create new ways to share responsibility, to support lifestyle needs of employees, and to provide flexible employee benefits and services (Kamerman and Kahn, 1987). Mathis and Jackson (1985) have pointed out that future managers will have to make more allowances for individual differences in people.

Admission to Professional Schools

GPA's and Medical College Admission Tests do not measure traits, such as interpersonal skills, empathy, and the ability to communicate with people, that are believed to be necessary to a good doctor. In fact, neither grades nor test scores are good predictors of success in medical school. For this reason, health professions schools do not use grades or test scores as the only, or major, criteria for accepting students. Admissions committees also look at personality, campus and community activities, work history, personal history and aspirations, and other traits. In light of this knowledge, a task force at the University of California at Davis recommended that a special program be instituted to admit disadvantaged students. Under this plan, a number of places would be reserved for consideration by a Special Admissions Committee composed primarily of minority medical faculty and staff. In 1970, eight students entered this program. The Davis faculty found the academic performance of these students satisfactory enough to expand the number.

In 1972, Alan Bakke, a White male, applied for admission to medical school. Because Bakke applied late, few regular places were open. The admission committee had set aside 16 of the 100 places for special admissions. Upon hearing of the Special Admissions Program, Bakke felt aggrieved that non-Whites were given special consideration (Stasz, 1981). He hired an attorney who successfully argued his case before the California Supreme Court. Bakke was admitted to the medical school at Davis. However, the University of California appealed the case to the U.S. Supreme Court, which affirmed the right of schools to take race into account in admissions and affirmed the commitment to erase racial inequality.

Bunzel (1988) notes that it is not unusual to be told by university officials that "special sensitivity" is shown to certain ethnic minority groups, and that membership in such a group is an "important factor" in the choice of a minority candidate over a White one who has better academic credentials. The same officials are reluctant to discuss the point at which "special sensitivity" becomes outright preference, or the limits to which they are willing to "stretch" the admission requirements to obtain the desired minority representation. Klitgaard (1985) states that admissions officers are conspicuously vague about policies of preferential admission. They prefer to point out the diversity they are creating. Diversity is open to different meanings and interpretations.

On the other hand, deans in many medical schools have a given number of "administrative" places in each class of entering students that are available for privileged individuals, for example, relatives of a state senator who has been a supporter of the school. Thus, the guardians of the boundaries of admission to medical and other health professions schools can "stretch" the boundaries for reasons other than ethnic diversity. Admission committees, however, usually try to adhere to quantitative criteria to make the management of admissions "easier" and "more defendable."

Interdisciplinary Groups/Programs/Care

A single health discipline or occupation rarely, if ever, meets all of most patients' needs. When health professionals from several disciplines attempt to work together in caring for patients or teaching students, the end product, hopefully, is better quality. The interdisciplinary process is more than the gathering of health professionals to discuss a patient. Each professional brackets his or her professional-discipline-identity and replaces it with the new identity of team member. This is what Goffman (1974) would regard as the ability to "break frame."

The act of bracketing is critical to the process of interdisciplinarity (Davis, 1987). As Davis explains, "each of us sits down with a willingness to allow others to change . . . this way the very best of all possible plans is agreed upon . . . ideally professional boundaries transcend and flow into each other much like a rainbow" (p. 1029). Individuals come together without territorial boundary needs to guide their roles and responsibilities, resulting in the highest form of care. Hospice care illustrates the process very well.

Factors that interfere with interdisciplinary care include:

- lack of personal commitment to the process
- lack of personal commitment to accepting the risk of bracketing one's professional role
- feelings of insecurity that are revealed in clear territorial boundary roles
- lack of shared values
- lack of skill in interpersonal interaction
- perceptions of threat from other team members
- instruction that presents a narrow view of other disciplines

Muldary (1983) notes that personnel can function in health care organizations for years and never get to know the persons in other roles. He states that this seems to be consistent with people's needs to survive in the organization so that they learn to conceal their real selves and project an image that conforms to normative expectations. If individuals are concerned with defending themselves in their roles, interpersonal trust is not encouraged. Muldary points out the curious paradox that while health professionals occupy roles that label them as trustworthy, trust does not characterize peer relationships within health care organizations.

Ducanis and Golin (1979) have studied interdisciplinary teams extensively. Their Interprofessional Perception Scale (IPS) yields data regarding how members of one profession view members of another, whether they think members of that profession agree or disagree with their view, and whether they understand that perception. The scale can also be used to indicate how subjects perceive their own profession and whether they think other professionals agree with or understand this perception.

These researchers measured the perceptions of physicians, nurses, and a variety of allied health professionals including physical therapists, medical technologists, nutritionists, respiratory therapists, occupational therapists, social workers, and child care workers. Nurses misunderstood the capabilities of the allied health professionals and most of the respondents stated that nurses and physicians did not know the competencies of allied health professionals.

In a revision of the IPS, Ducanis and Golin studied 115 health professionals including nurses, physical therapists, special education teachers, and rehabilitation counselors. While most of the respondents saw other professions encroaching on their territory to some degree, over 70 percent of the physicians indicated that their territory was being encroached upon. These researchers have also devised a process and instrument (Team Observation Protocol) for identifying participants in team discussions, the types of statements made by various professionals, and how a team reaches a decision.

Total Quality Management (TQM)

Most observers of health care readily admit that the present system of cost containment is futile, even in the short run. New dimensions need to be considered. Equally as important as the cost of care is the quality of services delivered. During this era of restrictions on government spending, cost shifting, and regulation of physician-patient relations, innovative plans are being proposed to improve quality. In the business sector, orientation toward changes based on customer (consumer) needs has been shown to lower operating costs, improve efficiencies, and increase profit margins (Miller and Milakovich, 1991). A recent survey of physicians and other health care providers revealed that 78 percent of the physicians, purchasers, and third-party payers, and 69 percent of the institutional providers, felt that quality improvement programs could reduce operating expenses by 20 to 40 percent (Miller and Milakovich, 1991).

Insurance companies, health maintenance organizations, preferred provider organizations, corporations with large medical bills, and government reimbursement agencies have supported efforts to encourage primary care providers to be more "businesslike." In addition, hospitals have recently begun to adopt and implement total quality care improvement systems based on business models (Milakovich, 1991).

Quality is often perceived as a fixed commodity that only health care professionals can define, rather than as a strategic mission shared by the entire organization. Health professionals are encouraged to design and implement total quality improvement systems capable of improving all aspects of quality care. A continuous commitment to client (patient) driven internal process improvement could begin to shift attitudes away from dependence on cost control and external regulations as the only means of achieving higher levels of quality.

Total quality care is a unique combination of applied modern high technology, access to facilities at reasonable costs, patient-centered, high quality primary and specialized clinical care, and low-tech holistic human healing skills (Milakovich, 1991). Before health care managers can deploy quality as a strategic management tool, a service-oriented quality culture must be created, and measures of clinical care must be integrated with financial, cost-control, and patient satisfaction measures. Creating a positive environment for total quality care requires a great degree of cross-functional coordination and vertical integration between medical, managerial, and support staffs. Equally important, total quality care must develop within the organization from the bottom up. Everyone must be included because the entire facility is subject to continuous improvement.

Before it is possible to realize total quality as a strategic management vision, the costs of poor quality must be acknowledged, measurement systems must be designed to accurately translate these costs, and team-based quality indicators must be established. The entire organization must be involved in the critical task of identifying the indicators to be monitored. Administrators must know how total quality management differs from other management strategies, reexamine annual employee merit review procedures to reward quality improvement efforts, include teams as units of analysis, emphasize extended patient satisfaction, provide incentives for training all employees, and develop patient-defined measures of quality.

Casalou (1991) notes that total quality management requires the breaking down of barriers between departments. Individuals from all the departments must be able to communicate freely. People can work in separate departments, but the goals of different departments cannot be in conflict.

In describing an effort to implement TQM in a 165 bed community hospital in Texas, Lynn (1991) stressed three major components: quality orientation, continuous process improvement, and total employee involvement. A hospital policy evolved that was dedicated to improving the quality of patient care. A process improvement approach, instituted in several areas of the hospital, improved the accuracy of patient billing, retained nurses, shortened the turnaround time in the emergency room, improved the promptness of medical record entries, and improved the quality of dietary service, discharge planning, and purchasing procedures. A survey was sent to former patients of the hospital twice a year to assess these areas. One hundred employees at the hospital voluntarily formed 15 improvement teams. Each team had a leader, facilitator, timekeeper, and recorder, and each member of the team had the opportunity to experience all of these roles. Preliminary results in the first three months showed the number of incomplete medical records to have dropped by 50 percent.

Candy and Crebert (1991) point out that breaking down barriers among disciplines is not easy. One of the most difficult adaptations required of the university graduate is the change from acting and learning as an individual to performing as a member of a group or team. In fact, university graduates are often undesirable employees because they have had "an unconscious training in anti-teamwork." These authors propose that our educational system employ a range of learning styles, such as self-directed learning and problem-based learning, to break down the stress on individual achievement, personal ambition, personal goals, and personal rewards. Some universities have implemented total quality management, e.g., Oregon State University, (Coate, 1990). TQM seems most easily applied within the service units of a university, such as the physical plant, personnel, library, admissions, and records. Assessing the quality of academic programs, faculty, and students is more complex. Early team performance is discouraged in academia; it is an individual's ability to compete successfully for grants, write peer-reviewed papers that which will be accepted for publication by prestigious journals, and become an established leader in one's profession that result in promotion, tenure, and merit pay increases.

Fairweather and Brown (1991) examined the dimensions of academic quality and suggested that three dimensions—size, resources, and accreditation—are best examined at the program level. Institutional-level indicators of these dimensions did not cluster with corresponding program-level measures, limiting their utility in assessing program quality. Results also show that "student quality" is complex. Institutional selectivity of students does not necessarily indicate program selectivity. Measures of prestige and faculty quality are closely tied to program measures. Instituting TQM in academic programs would not only be complex, but would be in direct opposition to current university culture and faculty freedom.

Quality Circles and Self-Directed Work Groups

Effective managers are now reintegrating work processes. They are delegating many of their traditional duties to small groups of frontline people, variously called high-performance teams, semi-autonomous teams, self-directed teams, work teams, new venture teams, quality circles, communication teams, task forces, or just plain teams. Teams have been established in many industries, such as General Motors, General Foods, General Electric, Pepsi-Cola, Hewlett-Packard, Honeywell, IBM and Xerox.

Teams may be temporary or permanent, specialized or crossfunctional, synonymous or auxiliary to the activities of natural work groups, conventionally supervised, or self-managed (Zenger *et al.,* 1991). Team management has become more responsive to the changing needs of the workforce and to the pressures of competition. The traditional manager must respond to a new environment by adding several new layers of leadership skills, developing self-motivated people, helping diverse people generate ideas, building self-managing teams, championing crossfunctional efforts, managing change, and sharing power.

Carr (1991) notes that empowered people are like gyroscopes—you set the direction and they function on their own. He points out that traditional organizations have interlocked power and dependence relationships. In a self-managed environment, power is shared and the emphasis is on working together to reach common goals. Successful organizations are usually empowering organizations. Managing in an empowering organization has many facets: managing alignment (to see that employees are clear about the goal and working toward it), managing coordination (to see that there is open communication and that resources are available to all components), managing the decision process (making certain everyone has input into decisions), managing continuous learning (to see that all employees have an opportunity to up-date their skills), and creating and maintaining trust (maintaining open dialogue and giving authority along with responsibility). Empowerment is an ongoing process.

Barry (1991) asks, "how should leadership be exercised in leaderless settings?" Most leadership theories are person-centered. There are two well-known group-centered leadership models. The Tannenbaum-Schmidt model focuses on centralizing decision-making within the group. At one extreme is the leader who dominates the group, and at the other extreme is the leader who permits group decisions within limits. Tannenbaum-Schmidt stresses the importance of focusing on the group's decision-making process and the social leadership roles which evolve, especially as these factors relate to management participation and conflict.

Blanchard's situational leadership model is concerned with how directive and socially centered group functions vary as a group matures. In the early phase of a group, commitment is high and task competence is low; leadership that is high in directiveness and low in supportiveness seems to work best. Conversely, a leadership style that is high in support and low in direction is more effective during the latter stages of a group when morale and competence are high.

Barry (1991) proposes a third type of self-managed team, the distributed leadership model. He notes that certain individual, task, and organizational variables can reduce a group's need for leadership; the need for formal leadership decreases when team members are able, experienced, trained and knowledgeable, when tasks are routine and results-driven, and when organizational processes emphasize high levels of formality, cohesiveness, inflexibility, and spatial distinction between workers (e.g., health care team in a burn center, rehabilitation or trauma center, or emergency room). When leadership is distributed, a collection of roles and behaviors can be split, shared, rotated, and used. Depending on which situation may arise, there may be multiple leaders and the active cultivation of new leaders. This type of self-directed team has been common in highly specialized areas of patient care. It is less common in primary care.

Goldberg and Pegels (1985) reviewed the experiences of five health care facilities that have been forerunners of the quality circle movement in the United States. Quality circles were introduced at the Henry Ford Hospital in Detroit in 1981. Six departments were selected as test areas: dietetics, general stores, housekeeping, computer services, occupational therapy, and the business office. Volunteers were solicited for quality circle membership in each of these departments. Interest among employees was high. After six months of operation, an evaluation revealed that employee morale, job satisfaction, and cooperation had improved. By 1982, the initial six circles had expanded to seventeen.

A senior manager at Children's Hospital Medical Center of Northern California in Oakland implemented quality circles in 1981, beginning with two circles, one in pharmacy and one in the research laboratory. Additional circles were planned in medical records, patient accounts, physical therapy, social services and engineering. Some problems addressed by the quality circles involved orienting new employees, prioritizing workloads, the quantity and quality of work measurements, procedures for message taking and updating telephone extension lists. In 1982, with the departure of the senior manager, the circle activities were transferred from human resources to industrial engineering. The hospital began a Total Quality Management Program in 1990.

St. Joseph's Hospital in Fort Wayne, Indiana implemented quality circles in 1981 with the formation of a hospital-wide steering committee. Quality circles were formed in nine departments—central supply, engineering, patient accounts, housekeeping, maintenance, medical records, laboratory, pharmacy, and medical-surgical nursing. The circles were requested initially to work on single problems to gain experience and ensure positive results. The most comprehensive early project, to improve organization and safety in nursing, electronic, and X-ray services, was undertaken by the quality engineers. By 1982, a total of 15 quality circles were functioning. A program in Total Quality Management was begun in 1990.

Barnes Hospital in St. Louis, Missouri, was one of the first hospitals to implement quality circles. Eight circles were established and, by 1982, a total of 33 quality circles were functioning. One problem in implementing quality circles has been the perception of the part-time facilitator as an "outsider." Department heads perceived the quality circle concept as having originated outside their own environment, not as something "owned" by them.

Lakeshore Mental Health Institute in Memphis began a quality circle program in 1981 with five circles. The circles worked on ways to reduce costs, improve work procedures, and improve the quality of patient care. An interdepartmental circle worked on several communication problems, resulting in improved scheduling of appointments, a more timely arrangement of transportation, and a centralized system for scheduling patient appointments.

Developing Health Care Teams—Constraints

Shortell (1982) notes that while health care professionals increasingly are trained to take a holistic view of patients, many do not take a holistic view of themselves as health care professionals. Health professionals tend to view each other in a segmented and instrumental manner. Each simply represents to the other a means of doing a job. When this perception of other professionals is coupled with differences in professional culture, it is far easier to understand patients than co-workers.

Proposals for change include joint nurse-physician management of patient care units, nurse involvement as voting members of hospital governing boards, and the development of voluntary nursing staff organizations paralleling that of the voluntary medical staff. Because of the hospital's demand for nurses, which consistently seems to outgrow the supply, nurses are in a particularly favorable economic position to press for these and related changes. Some attributes of Theory Z management, particularly consensual decision-making and developing holistic views of people, could facilitate changes in the roles of nurses and other health personnel with respect to sharing power and decision-making. However, for this to occur, physicians and administrators will have to "give up" some of their autonomy and professional elitism (Shortell, 1982).

The key question is whether health care managers are willing to place their careers in the service of values and willing to risk the possibility of new values, such as quality care. As Shortell points out, concern for quality involves more than managerial preference. It involves the development of a distinctive organizational philosophy and culture that is shared by all participants. This will require major shifts in professional boundaries as we now know them.

How Change Reshapes Boundaries

Environment typically is seen as everything outside the boundaries of an organization and as the major source of change. However, different parts of an organization may face different environments; hence, all change is not necessarily externally induced. Most likely, social change is a complex, ongoing interaction between forces internal and external to the organization (Glatter, 1989).

Sources of Change

Sathe (1985) observed that management can effect change by influencing behavior, by altering organizational culture, or by a combination of the two. Asay and Maciariello (1991) refer to the 4C's of management: control as promoting creativity, being a catalyst, securing contributions, and stimulating creativity. Greiner (1972) noted that the future of organizations may be determined less by outside events than by their own histories. He observed that the experiences of people within organizations change their perceptions of the effectiveness of their organizations, and he believed that these experiences eventually propel them into crisis situations that force change. Greiner noted that organizations appear to go through a series of evolutionary growth phases, each of which is punctuated by a crisis that requires a new form of leadership. Each crisis requires a solution before the organization can proceed to the next phase of growth. The stages, or phases, are: growth by creativity, growth by direction, growth by delegation, growth by coordination, and growth by collaboration.

Management Style and Change

Management is a dynamic, interpersonal activity that can be observed in the behavior styles of managers and subordinates. Crowe and his colleagues (1972) tested the assumption that managers accommodate their management style to that of their subordinates, irrespective of their own preferences: a democratic manager exposed to autocratic subordinates will tend to behave autocratically, whereas an autocratic manager exposed to democratic subordinates will become more democratic in his behavior. Through time, an autocratic style promotes passivity and dependence, while a democratic one stimulates initiative and self-reliance. Findings established that managers are as much a target of influence as they are a source of influence, supporting the view that it makes good sense to adapt one's leadership style to the constraints of a situation.

There is evidence to support the view that leaders with democratic styles are more likely than leaders with autocratic styles to have organizations that cope with change effectively. Employees in an organization form global beliefs concerning the extent to which the organization values their contributions and cares about their well-being. Perceived organizational support has been shown to reduce absenteeism (Eisenberger *et al.*, 1986). The relation between perceived organizational support and absenteeism is greater for employees with a strong exchange ideology than for those with a weak exchange ideology. These findings support the view that employees' commitment to an organization is strongly influenced by their perception of the organization's commitment to them. It has been found that a lack of involvement by employees can result in alienation, mismanagement, and low productivity (Simmons and Mares, 1983).

Leadership style is critical to organizations, especially those undergoing rapid and pervasive change. Some groups and individuals seize the opportunity to exert power or join groups that are perceived to be powerful. Such power plays, if successful, usually result in groups and individuals establishing rigid boundaries, and, as Häring (1975) states, a "selective conscience." Rigidly defined and limited roles make adaptation to change difficult for the organization and will, no doubt, impede completing tasks and reaching goals (Singer, *et al.,* 1975).

Employee Empowerment and Change

Empowerment is a means of achieving participative management. It is the mechanism by which responsibility is vested in teams or individuals. Involvement is the mechanism for ensuring appropriate input into decision-making. Thus, empowerment and involvement become the building blocks for participative management. Plunkett and Fournier (1991) point out that participative management involves learning to share information, share success, and manage failure. They stress that, in times of rapid change, it is important for workers to be knowledgeable and informed in order to adapt and to assist the organization for which they work to adapt. They describe a traditional power and information grid in a hospital where doctors and nurses have the greatest amount of power, and nurses have, in addition, a great amount of information. Nurse assistants have a great amount of information, but no power, and administrators have neither information nor power.

This type of power and information grid is no longer appropriate if hospitals are to survive. Plunkett and Fournier discuss the need for integrated and natural work teams, where information is shared by all who are responsible for the care of patients. The powerful hospitals are those which survive economically because they are known for high standards of patient care. Shortell (1985) outlines ten characteristics of high-performing health care organizations, one of which is their ability to stretch themselves. High-performing health care organizations develop overarching goals, which unite departments within the organization and tie the organization to the community. Healthy health care organizations are always in the process of change. No matter how good their current performance, they believe they can do better.

Excellent health care organizations have programs that emphasize interpersonal, technical, and management skills. They view all members, physicians, nurses, and others, as managers in varying degrees. They emphasize the manager-as-developer rather than the manager-as-master-technician approach. The manager-as-developer approach emphasizes leadership through the development of one's subordinates. The result is that subordinates' skill levels increase along with their confidence and commitment to the organization. This approach also makes available to the organization a rich array of management skills, more than any single manager can alone possess. As one CEO said, "We deliberately design our management positions so they cannot reasonably be filled by one person" (Shortell, 1985).

High-performing health care organizations not only respond to change, but are change makers (Shortell, 1985). A wide search of the environment, information processing, maximizing learning, taking risks, training managers to be developers, facilitating the flow of information, allowing decision-making at lower organizational levels, and creating a "congeniality of excellence," are all characteristics that help a healthy organization cope with uncertainty and change. As Shortell (p. 34) states, "In benign environments, almost everyone looks good . . . in more hostile environments poor management and poor clinical performance become transparent, and the truly outstanding organizations rise to the challenge."

Bennis (1987), in discussing indicators of an organization's health (effectiveness), states that the main challenge confronting today's organization is that of responding to changing conditions and to external stress. Most revealing about an organization's health is how it goes about the process of problem-solving. Bennis points out some parallels between the evaluation of an individual's mental health and that of an organization's health. Flexibility, adaptability, or the ability to change with changing internal and external circumstances is the key to maintaining an organization's health.

The Role of the Boundary Manager and Change

The boundary manager needs to manage while leading change. The boundary manager must neutralize the negative effects, and emphasize the positive effects, of change. In a sense, the boundary manager must create a neutral situation so that people affected by boundary changes will not spend a great deal of time debating the pluses and minuses of the old versus the new. The boundary manager must assist those affected by change to learn new tasks and responsibilities with ease and dispatch. The process of "unfreezing" the old and "re-freezing" the new must occur simultaneously to reduce anxiety about possible role losses and fears of

TABLE 6-1

Some Effects of Expanding or Retracting Boundaries in Health Disciplines

Expanding Boundaries	Retracting Boundaries
▼ Discipline becomes broad with blurred mission and goals	▼ Loss of power and prestige
▼ Risk of splinter groups forming	▼ Less visible and known to others
▼ More difficult to achieve consensus with diverse interests	▼ Encourages sub-specialization
▼ Competition between segments of discipline	▼ Scope of work narrow and threatened by change
▼ Strong leadership needed	▼ More difficult to recruit because discipline is less known and visible
▼ Difficult to keep abreast of expanding knowledge; encourages specialization	▼ Narrow focus and concerns of members
▼ Concern over depth of preparation	▼ Fortification of boundaries by strong credentials and membership requirements
▼ Increased "turf" battles to fight off boundary intrusions by overlapping interests of other groups	▼ Concern over member attrition; opportunities for professional growth limited

Source: John G. Bruhn

failure in the new situation. Boundary managers are front-line therapists or, as DePree (1989) would call them, "roving leaders" in an organization. They must be secure enough to deal with the insecurities of workers, while simultaneously keeping the organization moving forward.

Table 6-1 compares some of the consequences of expanding or retracting boundaries in health disciplines. Change always creates trade-offs. Since it is natural to resist change, the trade-offs will no doubt be viewed more often as negative than as positive by the affected persons. Establishing a new equilibrium is essential in keeping an organization viable. The boundary manager must be attuned to restoring equilibrium to an organization undergoing change.

In traditional health organizations, the boundary manager is the vice president, dean, department chair, or director of a unit. In health organizations, which are to be leaders, innovators and, indeed, survive in the future, every person has the potential of being a boundary manager. Administrators need to perfect their skills as participative managers, sharing their information and power.

REFERENCES

Altman, Stuart M, Brecher, Charles, Henderson, Mary G., and Thorpe, Kenneth E. (eds.): *Competition and Compassion: Conflicting Roles for Public Hospitals.* Ann Arbor, MI, Health Administration Press, 1989.

Anderson, Gerard F., Lave, Judith R., Russe, Catherine M. and Newuman, Patricia: *Providing Hospital Services: The Changing Financial Environment.* Baltimore, Md., Johns Hopkins University Press, 1989.

Asay, Lyal D., and Maciariello, Joseph A.: *Executive Leadership in Health Care.* San Francisco, Jossey-Bass, 1991.

Barry, David: Managing the bossless team: Lessons in distributed leadership. *Organizational Dynamics, 20,* 31–47, 1991.

Bennis, Warren G.: Toward a "truly" scientific management: The concept of organization health. In Schein, Edgar H. (ed.): *The Art of Managing Human Resources.* New York: Oxford, 1987.

Bunzel, John H.: Affirmative action admissions: How it "works" at U.C. Berkeley. *The Public Interest, 93:* 111–129, 1988.

Candy, P.C., and Crebert, R.G.: Ivory tower to concrete jungle: The difficult transition from the academy to the workplace as learning environments. *Journal of Higher Education, 62:* 570–592, 1991.

Carr, Clay: Managing self-managed workers. *Training and Development Journal, 45:* 37–42, 1991.

Casalou, Robert F.: Total quality management in health care. *Hospital and Health Services Administration, 36:* 136–146, 1991.

Coate, L. Edwin: Implementing total quality management in a university setting. Unpublished paper. Oregon State University, July, 1990.

Coile, Russell C., Jr.: *The New Medicine: Reshaping Medical Practice and Health Care Management.* Rockville, MD, Aspen, 1990.

Crowe, Bruce J., Bochner, Stephen, and Clark, Alfred W.: The effects of subordinates' behavior on managerial style. *Human Relations, 25:* 215–237, 1972.

Davis, Carol M.: Philosophical foundations of interdisciplinarity in caring for the elderly: Or, the willingness to change your mind. *Proceedings, Book II, Tenth International Congress of the World Federation for Physical Therapy.* Sydney, Australia, May 17–22, 1987.

De Pree, Max: *Leadership is an Art.* New York, Dell, 1989.

Ducanis, Alex J., and Golin, Anne K.: *The Interdisciplinary Health Care Team: A Handbook.* Germantown, MD, Aspen, 1979.

Eisenberger, Robert, Huntington, Robin, Hutchinson, Steven, and Sowa, Debra: Perceived organizational support, *Journal of Applied Psychology, 71:* 500–507, 1986.

Epstein, Cynthia F.: *Woman's Place.* Berkeley, CA, University of California Press, 1970.

Epstein, Cynthia F.: *Women in Law.* New York, Basic Books, 1981.

Fairweather, James S. and Brown, Dennis F.: Dimensions of academic program quality. *The Review of Higher Education, 14:* 155–176, 1991.

Glatter, Ron (ed.): *Educational Institutions and Their Environments: Managing Boundaries.* Philadelphia, Open University Press, 1989.

Glazer, Nathan: The affirmative action stalemate. *The Public Interest, 90:* 99–114, 1988.

Glazer, Nathan: Affirmative action as a remedy for discrimination. *American Behavioral Scientist, 28:* 829–841, 1985.

Goffman, Irving.: *Frame Analysis.* Cambridge, MA, Harvard University Press, 1974.

Goldberg, Alvin M., and Pegels, C. Carl: *Quality Circles in Health Care Facilities: A Model for Excellence.* Rockville, MD, Aspen, 1985.

Greiner, Larry E.: Evolution and revolution as organizations grow. *Harvard Business Review, 50:* 37–46, 1972.

Häring, Bernard: *Ethics of Manipulation.* New York, Seabury Press, 1975.

Jamieson, David, and O'Mara, Julie: *Managing Workforce 2000.* San Francisco, Jossey-Bass, 1991.

Kadushin, Alfred: Men in a woman's profession, *Social Work, 21:* 440–447, 1976.

Kamerman, Sheila B. and Kahn, Alfred J.: *The Responsive Workplace.* New York: Columbia University Press, 1987.

Kanter, Rosabeth Moss: *When Giants Learn to Dance.* New York, Simon & Schuster, 1989.

Klitgaard, Robert: *Choosing Elites.* New York, Basic Books, 1985.

Lewis, Irving J. and Sheps, Cecil G. *The Sick Citadel.* Cambridge, MA, Oelgeschlager, Gunn and Hain, 1983.

Lindorff, Dave: *Marketplace Medicine.* New York, Bantam Books, 1992.

Lynch, Frederick R: *Invisible Victims: White Males and the Crisis of Affirmative Action.* New York, Greenwood Press, 1989.

Lynn, Monty L.: Deming's quality principles: A health care application. *Hospital and Health Services Administration, 36:* 111–120, 1991.

Mathis, Robert L., and Jackson, John H.: *Personnel Human Resource Management.* 4th edition. New York, West, 1985.

Milakovich, Michael E.: Creating a total quality health care environment. *Health Care Management Review, 16:* 9–20, 1991.

Miller, Jack B., and Milakovich, Michael E.: Improving access to health care through total quality management. *Quality Assurance and Utilization Review, 6:* 138–141, 1991.

Muldary, Thomas W.: *Interpersonal Relations for Health Professionals: A Social Skills Approach.* New York, Macmillan Co., 1983.

Norman, Geoffrey R.: Problem-solving skills, solving problems and problem-based learning. *Medical Education, 22:* 279–286, 1988.

Norman, Geoffrey R., and Schmidt, Henk G.: The psychological basis of problem-based learning: A review of the evidence. *Academic Medicine, 67*(9): 557–565, 1992.

Odiorne, George S.: *The Change Resisters.* Englewood Cliffs, NJ, Prentice-Hall, 1981.

Plunkett, Lorne, and Fournier, Robert: *Participative Management: Implementing Empowerment.* New York, Wiley, 1991.

Rogers, David E.: *American Medicine: Challenge for the 1980s.* Cambridge, MA, Ballinger, 1978.

Sathe, Vijay: *Culture and Related Corporate Realities.* Homewood, IL, Dow Jones-Irwin, 1985.

Schein, Edgar H.: The mechanisms of change. In Bennis, Warren G., Benne, Kenneth D., and Chin, Robert (eds.): *The Planning of Change.* 2nd edition. New York, Holt, Rinehart and Winston, 1969.

Schreiber, Carol Tropp: *Changing Places: Men and Women in Transitional Occupations.* Cambridge, MA, MIT Press, 1979.

Shortell, Stephen M.: High-performing health care organizations: Guidelines for the pursuit of excellence. *Hospital & Health Sciences Administration, 30:* 8–35, 1985.

Shortell, Steven M.: Theory Z: Implications and relevance for health care management. *Health Care Management Review, 7:* 7–21, 1982.

Simmons, John, and Mares, William: *Working Together.* New York, Alfred A. Knopf, 1983.

Singer, David, Astrachan, Boris M., Gould, Laurence J., and Klein, Edward B.: Boundary management in psychological work with groups. *Journal of Applied Behavioral Science, 11:* 137–176, 1975.

Stasz, Clarice: *The American Nightmare.* New York, Schocken, 1981.

Stemmler, Edward J.: The medical school—where does it go from here? *Academic Medicine, 64*(4): 182–185, 1989.

Szasz, George: Interprofessional education in the health sciences. *Milbank Memorial Fund Quarterly, 47*(4) (Part 1): 449–475, 1969.

Walton, Henry J., and Matthews, M.B.: Essentials of problem-based learning. *Medical Education, 23:* 542–558, 1989.

Wilson, Marjorie Price, Knapp, R.M., and Jones, A.B.: The growing managerial imperative of the academic medical center. In Levey, S., and McCarthy, T. (eds.): *Health Management for Tomorrow.* Philadelphia, J.B. Lippincott, 1980.

Wilson, Marjorie Price, and McLaughlin, Curtis P.: *Leadership and Management in Academic Medicine.* San Francisco, Jossey-Bass, 1984.

Zenger, John H., Musselwhite, Ed, Hurson, Kathleen, and Perrin, Craig: Leadership in a team environment. *Training and Development Journal, 45:* 47–52. 1991.

Zuckerman, Harriet, Cole, Jonathan R., and Bruer, John T. (eds.): *The Outer Circle: Women in the Scientific Community.* New York, W.W. Norton, 1991.

Chapter 7

MANAGING BOUNDARY
DIVERSITY AND CHANGE

Boundaries really exist only in our mind
Ernest Hartmann (1991)

Boundaries are the means we use to get some people together and keep others apart. While boundaries create conflict, they also provide structure and order for individuals as well as organizations. Lawrence (1979) has stated:

> Boundaries are necessary for human beings to relate not only to each other but through their institutions. If there are no boundaries, relatedness and relationships are impossible because we become one; lost in each other, lost in institutions, lost in societies. At the same time, it is readily recognized that boundaries can be used and experienced as impregnable barriers. Both the wish for no boundaries and the desire to remain totally imprisoned within a boundary are expressions of "madness," as there is no desire to distinguish between fantasy and reality (p. 16).

Non-physical boundaries are perceptual and, therefore, provide a filtering function. Boundaries screen inputs and outputs. Boundaries are barriers to the flow of energy, material, and information. Frequently, boundaries homogenize the inputs and filter the outputs so that individuals and organizations can deal with their environments more effectively. Boundaries also provide a degree of autonomy and independence from the intrusion of environmental influences. The filtering and buffering functions of boundaries are important for maintaining autonomy (Kast and Rosenzweig, 1985). The major function of boundary managers is to maintain the relative autonomy of all boundary parties while orchestrating their different talents to successfully accomplish common goals.

A boundary manager is a gatekeeper, a person who possesses much of the magic that makes collaboration and the crossing of boundaries work. The boundary manager orchestrates the precise mixture of roles needed to bring about a desired outcome. Division chiefs, department chairs, deans, and vice presidents in academic health science centers are boundary managers. They arbitrate the interests of students, faculty, and administration within and between their academic units. In essence, boundary managers attempt to maintain a balance within a system and between their system and the external environment. The style of management used to accomplish this balance involves the interaction of personalities, personal values, and perceptions.

It is important that boundary managers be given feedback about how effective they are in managing their boundaries. Faculty and student complaints can provide some insight into their effectiveness, but the effectiveness of boundary management should not be assessed according to how vocal or silent the constituents are. Employees' attitudes and behavior, which intrude upon or shape an organization's mission, are important. In the case of health care organizations, the effectiveness and excellence of client services also are important. In a medical school, the Chair of Medicine cannot be satisfied because the trainees and faculty are happy. The feelings of the surgeons, nurses, and allied health personnel, as well as those of the patients who are treated at the health science center, also are important. Boundary managers must have continual feedback as their "systems" are in constant flux. Managers should learn how to orchestrate personalities and resources so that effective collaboration may occur in their domain. Sometimes individuals inhibit collaboration, but usually, several factors interact to create a pattern of lack of cooperation or collaboration. Managers should explore options that can minimize deficits or problems and maximize available strengths.

Boundary managers cannot have vested interests. They must be eclectic and view the systems they manage through the effective functioning of their parts. Parts need to be repaired or changed to fine tune the system. This is a win/win approach to managing boundaries and is more likely than a disruptive win/lose approach to keep the system in relative balance (Covey, 1990). The terms, win/win and win/lose, which come from Berne's (1964) investigation of the "little" games we play with each other, in which there are usually winners and losers, aptly apply to boundary management. A win/win solution or resolution of a boundary conflict denotes a "good game," in which both parties or groups are winners. On the other hand, a win/lose approach to managing boundaries implies that one party or group has "done something wrong." A corrective management philosophy does not encourage the improvement of interrelationships.

Boundary management is not a state or trait, it is a process of perfecting the interrelationships between perceptions, personal values, and management style, which are changed and modified by intervention and experience. Continual direct and supportive feedback lets boundary managers know what they do well and what they need to improve.

In addition to receiving feedback from their immediate environments about the current functioning of their organizations, boundary managers need to be able to view emerging changes in the environment with vision and imagination. Health professions and health care institutions are in the grip of continuing, powerful forces, which will inevitably result in massive changes in resources and demands, and will greatly alter present boundaries. Employees of an organization often are unaware of the strength of the forces for change, and reluctant to respond to the need for change. Managers must try to educate their constituencies about forthcoming changes and prepare their organizations for future challenges.

Boundaries and Perceptions

People construct boundaries through their perceptions. Because perceptions arise from personal value systems, boundaries are not perceived by everyone in the same way. A boundary perceived by one person to be a fence may be perceived by another to be a wall. Indeed, perceptions of the types of boundaries needed, where they should be located, and their degree of permeability vary according to the value system of the perceiver. Sturgess (1991) has said, "Borders almost inevitably create conflict and tension. This is because it is almost impossible to define boundaries perfectly. . . . Given that there will always be territorial fights at the margin, the location of the fenceline determines just what those territorial fights are going to be about" (p. 12). Since personal value systems influence how boundaries are perceived, any boundary conflict involves personal values.

Of special concern in this book are occupational boundaries in the health professions. Changes in professional boundaries in the health professions usually are resisted strongly because they involve crossing levels of education and training. Higher-status professionals, who have made the greater investment in education and training, are unwilling to share responsibilities with lower-level professionals because they want both economic and career rewards from their investment (Karasek and Theorell, 1990). Flexibility might be increased if the higher-status group did not fear loss. The source of most boundary conflicts is the perception that one group will lose autonomy, power, status, prestige, income, or identity.

Stevens (1991) notes that the question in most health care turf wars is "who is more qualified and therefore should be responsible to do a particular task?" The implied message is, "*I* am more qualified than *you* to manage this task." Turf wars most commonly occur within the same discipline or between different disciplines. However, related disciplines can form coalitions for protection against "outside" groups. Turf wars generally erupt because involved parties are insecure about their values, unable to see the value of others who have different backgrounds but similar talents, or unable to understand or appreciate the contributions of individuals who are seen as adversaries. While there are numerous examples of divisiveness among groups, difficult circumstances can bring about innovations that cross disciplinary boundaries. The shortage of some types of health personnel, and the issue of cost containment, have led some hospitals, especially smaller, rural hospitals, to employ multiskilled practitioners. While multiskilled practitioners are not new, there are now a greater number and variety of formal programs that prepare multiskilled health practitioners. In a national survey of 546 hospitals using multiskilled workers, flexibility and efficiency, cost effectiveness, and employee satisfaction were the major reasons cited for employing multiskilled workers. It is noteworthy that hospitals using multiskilled workers reported that certain behavioral and personality traits enable these workers to be effective—adaptability, flexibility, innovative, creative, self-directed, and people-oriented. Several hospitals indicated that middle-aged employees performed better in multiskilled jobs than younger and older employees, and that higher level professionals had more difficulty accepting job responsibilities requiring additional skills than did lower level professionals (Vaughan and Bamberg, 1989). It could be concluded that age and status influence the perception of boundaries and the willingness to cross them.

Types of Boundary Structures

Boundaries can be structured in four general ways: closed, compact, porous, and open.

Individuals may experience a variety of types of boundaries depending upon the situation; how these individuals perceive the boundaries is a dimension of their personalities (Hartmann, 1991). Some boundaries are

FIGURE 7-1
Types of Boundary Structures

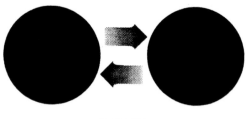

CLOSED

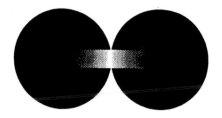

COMPACT

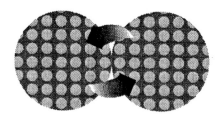

POROUS

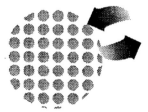

OPEN

Source: John G. Bruhn

clear, others are less distinct. And, our perceptions of boundaries can change. How we perceive boundaries is in our minds.

Some of the key characteristics of boundary types are listed in Table 7-1. Closed boundaries are the most dramatic because they are exclusionary and maintain strict control over who can cross the boundary line. The world is filled with examples of turf wars that erupted because people crossed closed boundaries or attempted to close once open boundries. Dramatic examples include the ethnic warfare between Serbians, Croatians, and Muslim factions in what was formerly Yugoslavia, the struggle of Blacks to obtain equality in South Africa, and the historical, territorial struggles between numerous groups in the Middle East.

Homogeneity is a primary characteristic of closed boundaries. Homogeneity ensures a high degree of control over the interests of specific groups, regulating change from within while fending off the external forces of change that impinge upon its boundaries. Groups and organizations that maintain closed boundaries have strict membership requirements and take pride in their autonomy. Closed boundary groups and organizations are often very powerful because they are able to maintain strict control over their purposes and missions, hence their efforts are not diluted by competing interests. However, homogeneity in membership and exclusionary rules also promote varying degrees of elitism. Table 7-1 gives some examples of health professional groups that are largely closed.

A second type of boundary structure, which is compact in nature, has limits and restrictions, but interacts with other groups and organizations. It is not as autonomous as the closed boundary, but, nonetheless, is tightly controlled. Nursing, occupational therapy, and physical therapy are independent disciplines, yet each must interact with physicians and other health professionals to accomplish its mission. Groups and organizations in the health arena that have compact boundaries usually are less powerful and less prestigious than are disciplines with closed boundaries.

A third type of boundary structure is porous. The key characteristics of porous boundaries are flexibility and adaptability. Porous boundary structures are characteristic of health care teams, where information exchange and a diverse set of skills are necessary for solving problems. Boundaries separating disciplines in health care teams must be fluid because not all disciplines have the necessary expertise for solving complex problems. Increasingly, porous boundaries are needed in caring for the chronically ill, for the disabled, and for victims of physical and psychological trauma.

TABLE 7-1
Some Characteristics of Boundary Types

Types of Boundaries	Characteristics	Examples
CLOSED	• control and decision-making centralized • roles and mission clear and limited • interaction with others formal and task-centered • autonomous, private • leadership is highly protective of group • minimal change from within group	• Surgery • Cardiology • Pathology • Dentistry • Emergency room • Anatomy • Anesthesiology
COMPACT	• leadership exerts control with purposeful interaction • interaction, teamwork controlled • credentials important and influence types of interaction • can be autonomous • roles and mission clear within group • attempt to control effects of external change	• Psychiatry • Nursing • Physical therapy • Occupational therapy • Psychology • Pharmacy
POROUS	• interaction with others encouraged • reciprocal give and take important to succeed • leadership is secure enough to delegate limited authority • adaptability to change important • team work appropriate • larger purpose supercedes individual roles and successes • input from outside welcomed but screened	• Social work • Physician's Assistants • Infectious disease specialists • Medical Records • Rehabilitation teams • Cancer center
OPEN	• control and decision-making largely de-centralized • roles and mission broad, flexible, changing • high degree of dependence on other disciplines • interaction with others informal and mixed purpose • leadership may defer to community, client or others for direction • change is constant and often rapid	• Community medicine • Health education • Preventive medicine • Hospital administration

Source: John G. Bruhn

Open boundaries are the fourth type of boundary structure. Groups and organizations in the health professions with open boundaries often lack prestige because they are broad in scope and continually are undergoing varying degrees of change. It is impossible to be "the expert" in an open boundary organization because of the expanse of knowledge and skills needed. In addition, there are fewer "givens" in open boundary organizations. There is a need to be proactive to anticipate and plan for the needed expertise. In this sense, open boundary groups and organizations are at the opposite end of the spectrum from closed boundary groups and organizations. City and county health departments are an example of open boundary organizations. Their mission includes the full spectrum of primary care. They may intervene in the case of individuals, e.g., providing primary care to pregnant women, or of an entire community, e.g., administering mass vaccinations against dangerous viruses.

Boundary Structures and Management Styles

The boundary structure of a group or organization influences its leadership and management styles. Leadership and management styles, in turn, help to maintain the predominate boundary structure of the group or organization. Table 7-2 shows the relationships between styles of leadership and styles of managing different types of boundaries. Leadership styles extend along a continuum from autocratic, authoritarian, and supervisory, at one extreme, to laissez-faire, nondirective, and permissive, at the other. A mixture of these styles, referred to as "democratic," represents the middle ground. Groups and organizations with closed and compact boundaries are likely to have leaders and managers who are authoritative, directive, and concerned with control. These leaders and managers are strong protectors of their boundaries and may be aggressors if new opportunities to acquire additional territory should arise. Permissive and nondirective leaders and managers are likely to be found in groups and organizations with porous and open boundaries. They encourage their constituents to participate in decision-making and delegate authority and responsibility to them. These leaders and managers most often will negotiate and arbitrate boundary disputes.

Following are a number of examples of problem situations that relate to misunderstandings or poor management of boundary issues.

TABLE 7-2

Relationships Between Styles of Leadership and Management

	LEADERSHIP STYLE						
	Laissez-faire	Nondirective	Permissive	Democratic	Supervisory	Authoritarian	Autocratic
Decision-making Style	Participative, Group-centered			Consultive		Authoritative, Directive	
General Management Style		Delegate		Process-oriented		Control	
Boundary Structure Type		Open, Porous		Team-oriented		Compact, Closed	
Boundary Management Style		Permissive, Negotiator/Arbitrator		Mixed		Protector, Aggressor/Defender	

Source: John G. Bruhn

Example 1
Security At All Costs

Department A in a medical school in a large health science center has a long history. When the department was founded, 75 years ago, the mission was rather simple and straightforward—to teach medical students about preventive medicine. In those days, preventive medicine focused primarily on infectious disease epidemiology and environmental health. Over time, the mission of the department has changed only slightly. The required course, taught to second year medical students, was never popular among the students as it was considered to be "common sense." Failure to pass the course did not threaten one's survival in medical school. The course competed with basic science courses for students' study time. Therefore, lectures were poorly attended despite the faculty's attempt to revise the course yearly on the basis of student evaluations. The course was taught in lecture format and each of the department's four divisions had a separate section of the course. Students complained that the course was not integrated and not clinically relevant.

The department was not highly regarded among other departments in the medical school for many reasons, including the lack of clinical involvement of the faculty and the lack of leadership by the department in the area of preventive medicine. As preventive medicine became more important in research and teaching, the department sought to revise its mission. However, the faculty in the department resisted a brief, concise mission statement in favor of one that was broad enough to encompass the interests of the four departmental units. There have been attempts to involve selected faculty in other departments to teach in the medical student course, but there is a reluctance to involve too many "outside lecturers" lest other departments "take over" the course.

The departmental faculty have remained quite stable, with some turnover among younger, untenured faculty members. The division chiefs have been in place for years, many with funded research projects; therefore, they have a great deal of autonomy and resist efforts to alter the structure within the department. There have been three chairs of the department in the last five years. One chair was ousted because of faculty opposition to his management style. Two other chairs have attempted to update the departmental mission, revamp the medical student course, and involve faculty in other departments, e.g., Family Medicine, Pediatrics, in teaching in the department. Medical students have offered input into making their course more interesting and relevant. Yet, faculty members in the department have resisted changes.

The Dean of Medicine, due in part to pressure from basic science departments facing budget cuts, appointed a study committee to suggest alternative options for Department A. Study committees had made recommendations in the past. Options ranged from closing the department to consolidating it with another relevant department. Outside consultants had offered recommendations over the past several years. Yet, the department survives with its rigid, closed boundaries and lack of a meaningful departmental mission. It is likely that as long as financial resources do not require that Department A be supported from resources which would go to other departments, there will not be pressure to "do something about Department A" from faculty members outside the department. Eventually, Department A will change as senior tenured faculty members retire. This example illustrates how secure closed boundaries can be and how difficult it is to open them to new opportunities.

Example 1, "Security at All Costs," describes a department in a medical school that has a broad mission and should have open boundaries. However, the department is comprised of several strong interest groups led by senior faculty members who carefully control the boundaries of their groups. Hence, there is no teamwork within the department, and indeed, frequent personality conflicts and open competition for group resources. The department is perceived externally as fragmented, divisive, non-productive, and contributing little to the university's mission. In this situation, it is unlikely the department will "open up" until senior faculty in leadership positions leave or retire.

Example 2
Control and Grow

College B, in a comprehensive university, has grown and prospered with new degree programs in nursing and allied health, and over 10 million dollars in research and program funding. Dean Smith is popular among the faculty, is aggressive in seeking new opportunities for the college to grow, and prides herself in knowing what is going on in all aspects of the college's activities. While the college's programs involve public schools, hospitals, community agencies, and other organizations in its outreach, the boundaries remain under the tight control and supervision of Dean Smith.

The college budget has had a position for an Associate Dean, which has remained unfilled, for three years. Dean Smith complains about her workload and long work hours. Her supervisor has strongly encouraged her to fill the Associate Dean position so that she can have some help. A search committee was appointed by Dean Smith, but the process was so slow, finalists had to commit themselves to other jobs. Dean Smith sees a young faculty member in the college as a "good" Associate Dean when she receives tenure. It is obvious that Dean Smith does not want an Associate Dean. She does not want to share power, and enjoys the accolades she receives for her many accomplishments.

Directors who are hired to implement the grants the college has successfully acquired are finding that Dean Smith will not relinquish authority to them.

When Dean Smith is out of town, project directors find themselves in limbo with respect to signatures on personnel actions and expenditures. Dean Smith complains about the lack of progress on the projects and the project directors are becoming frustrated with their lack of autonomy. The project directors see Dean Smith's control as a lack of trust in their abilities.

While the boundaries between the college and the community are quite porous, the boundaries within the college are carefully controlled. Dean Smith says that she is a developer of people and a team player and does not understand why the project directors are unhappy. She does not see herself as a controlling person.

Example 2, "Control and Grow," is an example of a Dean who has successfully expanded the boundaries of her organization, takes pride in knowing what is going on in all aspects of the organization, and resists delegating authority while complaining that she is overworked and underpaid. The Dean's unwillingness to recruit additional administrators and senior faculty permits her to maintain prominence in the organization and enjoy the accolades of her success. Unfortunately, the success of the organization has grown dependent upon a strong leader and, with her departure, is certain to suffer a loss of morale, a feeling of uncertainty, lack of direction, and a high degree of staff and faculty turnover. Leaders and managers who focus all of their efforts on the growth of their organization to the exclusion of developing their members perpetuate a destructive dependence on meeting their own personal needs.

Example 3
Collaborate, But Control

School C, in a large health science center, had worked out a collaborative agreement to extend programs in physical and occupational therapy to a university in an area of the state with a predominantly Hispanic population, which has a severe shortage of therapists. The state legislature funded this special initiative in School C's budget. School C and the university both agreed that after six years the university would be in a position to apply for its own accreditation, and funding would go directly to the university. School C worked very closely with the university in planning and designing the teaching laboratories, recruiting faculty, ordering equipment, and discussing details of faculty evaluation, promotion, and student recruitment. The students and faculty would be under the control of School C initially, students would pay tuition to School C, and faculty would be on School C's payroll. All went smoothly until the Registrar at School C's campus became involved in the collection of student fees. To make it convenient for students, the university proposed that students participate in the registration at the university, pay their fees, and the university would return tuition to School C's campus and retain the ancillary fees so students could have library privileges, student health services, etc. The Registrar at School C's campus would have no part of this arrangement. He insisted that the students in these two programs register and pay fees to his campus and that he would return the student fees to the university. Indeed, the Registrar proposed that he would dispatch a representative from his office to fly to the university site to register the students and collect the tuition and fees each semester. This unique collaborative program, which had smoothly surmounted the expected hurdles, was complicated by the need for the Registrar to retain control of the registration process. Officials at the university smiled and commented, "He doesn't trust us!"

Example 3, "Collaborate, but Control," illustrates a situation of porous boundaries. A university extends its boundaries to offer needed programs at a sister campus. Within this successful collaborative venture, the Registrar at the extending university exerts his power to collect student fees and protect himself from liability and criticism related to possible problems in the registration process of students from "his university." This example shows that even porous boundaries have their limits.

Example 4
It's Everyone's Problem, But No One's Responsibility

Sometimes a problem can be so pervasive that it crosses all professional boundaries. Such is the case of AIDS. As the epidemic grew in numbers and effects over the past decade, hospitals, in particular, were inundated with increasing numbers of very sick people. Many of the people with AIDS who sought medical care had no health insurance, no jobs or income, and were cared for as indigent patients. Health Science Center D was such a source of care. In the early days of the epidemic, most AIDS patients at this center were seen by faculty from the Division of Infectious Diseases. As the numbers grew, there were insufficient faculty to see all of the confirmed or suspected cases of AIDS. AIDS patients filled the majority of beds under the control of Internal Medicine. The Chair of Medicine complained that medical students were unable to see a variety of medical problems since AIDS patients were filling all available beds. There was no attempt by university leaders to draw up a policy on how employees, students, or faculty who contracted AIDS would be treated. The Department of Preventive Medicine had no initiatives, on or off campus, in education or research on AIDS. There was a general hands-off attitude about the problem despite cries for help from the infectious diseases faculty and hospital administrators who feared that the university hospital might get a reputation as an AIDS hospital. The hospital CEO was especially concerned that the large number of AIDS patients might dissuade other patients from seeking care there.

The local health department established an HIV clinic in the community where people could be tested and counseled anonymously. Several employees, students, and faculty died from AIDS, and a few students who were learning to draw blood got finger sticks, all of which raised the level of fear and anxiety on the campus. A group of faculty approached the administration to request that a study committee be formed to outline campus policy and programs needed to deal with the epidemic. The committee met over a period of several months and sent a report to the President with recommendations. There was no follow-up on the report.

The infectious diseases faculty obtained help from volunteer faculty, fellows in medicine, and student physician's assistants in seeing the growing number of patients. The director of the Division of Infectious Diseases was entrepreneurial in obtaining grants from drug companies and, thereby, was able to hire additional help. The director and the Dean of one of the schools formed a campus-community committee to explore the possibility of establishing a hospice. The committee formed a speaker's bureau and actively conducted AIDS education in the community. The committee was never formally acknowledged by the leadership of the health science center. The committee has struggled to stay alive by holding fund-raising events and obtaining grants from the state Department of Health.

AIDS is everybody's problem since it pervades all areas of the world and all segments of society. While AIDS is a medical problem, its origin is non-medical. It's a problem like suicide, drug addiction, alcoholism, and human abuse—all of which have health effects—yet the leadership for education and prevention of these problems, as well as of AIDS, has had to come largely from outside the boundaries of the health care system.

Example 4, "It's Everyone's Problem, But No One's Responsibility" describes the reluctance of the administration of a health science center to provide leadership in providing care to AIDS patients even though the complexity of AIDS crossed the boundaries of all the center's disciplines. The administration feared the possibility that the institution might be stigmatized, discouraging other types of patients from seeking care there. These leaders and managers did not want to construct boundaries that would give shape and direction to more effective coping with an open boundary disease. In such a situation, existing resources become dissipated by trying to meet too many needs and all parties suffer.

Managing Multi-Level Boundaries in Complex Organizations

Schneider (1991) has discussed the management of boundaries at different levels of analysis, e.g. individual, family, group, and organizational. The process of managing boundaries in complex organizations requires that the manager be able to differentiate and integrate the various levels to work toward accomplishing the organization's mission. Managers face a crucial dilemma in determining how to maximize a sense of identity and autonomy in individuals and groups, yet maintain the interdependence, integration, and efficiency necessary to the organization if it is to function as an integrated whole. As Schneider (1991) points out, organizations need appropriate levels of differentiation and integration. This requires that boundaries be firm, yet flexible and that managers have the ability to manage the paradoxes and dilemmas that result. Example 5, "The Unappreciated Gift," illustrates the complexities of managing many different boundary levels in an organization.

Example 5
The Unappreciated Gift

University E, a growing and evolving medium-sized university, saw as its future mission the development of undergraduate and graduate programs in the health professions. The need for health professionals in this geographic area, interest on the part of local practicing health professionals, clinical ties with a regional university health center, and support from state legislators from the area all made this broad mission of the university realistic. The university's development board had been successful in raising corporate and other funds for new ventures. A member of this board, a well-known local physician, was also medical director of an international hospital chain, which was desirous of tapping into markets of needed health manpower to supply its hospitals. The local physician was the appropriate link with the hospital corporation for obtaining a donation to establish and equip the necessary laboratories to institute two extension training programs in allied health from a sister university.

All parties had their expectations of this cooperative alliance. University E saw the hospital corporation as a possible source of future support in establishing other health programs, the local physician gained recognition for helping his community train needed health manpower and helping his corporation obtain future professionals, the sister university saw the extension of their programs into a manpower shortage area as a means of helping the state cope with health manpower needs and obtaining recognition for this effort, and the university CEO saw this effort as a coup for the university's status and growth.

Despite their different expectations, the individual efforts of the various parties culminated with the construction of the new laboratory facilities for training the health manpower needed in this city. All individuals and groups would benefit in some way.

The time came for the university CEO to receive the check from the hospital corporation. All parties were invited to a luncheon at which the check would be handed over to the university. Television and newspaper coverage were arranged. The event appeared to go like clockwork. But when the newspaper story came out, there was no mention or picture of the local physician on the university development board who had arranged for the gift. The feature article, written by an inexperienced young writer who knew little about the evolution of the program or its intended purpose, gave only cursory mention to the hospital corporation. Instead, the article focused on explaining the health programs. CEO's of other local hospitals were pictured and mentioned. The hospital corporation's intention of using the press article for publicity was thwarted. The angry local doctor wrote to the university CEO resigning from the development board and distancing himself from future fund raising efforts between the university and the corporation. The local physician expected a letter of apology from the university CEO, but the CEO responded by having the university development officer smooth the physician's ruffled feathers. The costs to the university were potentially great; the development officer had been discussing a large donation to the university with this physician and his wife. When the members of the development board heard of this physician's resignation, they began taking sides and could not understand the CEO's reluctance to apologize. Individual boundaries became group boundaries and groups, in turn, became aligned against the university.

An uninvolved friend of the physician was told about this state of affairs by the development officer. At a luncheon meeting, the development officer, physician, and his friend fully discussed the entire affair. The development officer and the physician's friend asked the physician to reconsider his resignation. The university CEO, who was out of town and unavailable at the time of the meeting, finally decided to personally apologize to the physician. The physician agreed to withdraw his resignation from the development board. The dedication of the new laboratories was planned for the following month, at which time the physician, his contributions, and those of the corporation would be highlighted.

This example shows the complexities of simultaneously managing boundaries at many levels. The manager is the key to the type and speed of intervention in resolving conflicts. Neglected and unresolved boundaries can damage organizations immeasurably.

Example 6
Going Around the Boss

A faculty member in a university made an appointment to see the Vice President for Academic Affairs to present some innovative ideas for using technology in teaching. The Vice President directed the faculty member to various persons on and off campus who could help to plan and, possibly, implement these ideas. The faculty member made a second appointment for herself and two other persons, who, she said, had greater technological expertise than she did. They presented a budget for new equipment and a plan for space for this new venture.

The Vice President discovered that these plans were being devised without the knowledge or consent of the Department Chair. He informed the faculty member that he would not be a part of any future meetings unless the Department Chair were present. The Vice President then briefed the Department Chair and told him that any future meetings or actions would have to be initiated by him.

The Department Chair and the faculty member were the only two tenured, senior faculty in the Department. The Vice President learned that they had not worked together, and, indeed, had barely spoken to one another, since the Department Chair had been chosen over the opposition of the faculty member.

While people in organizations tend to "go around" others when they feel blocked or stymied, their motive also may be to point out to others the ineffectiveness of their boss. This "power play" involves transgressing boundaries and mobilizing someone high in the organizational hierarchy to intervene and either construct new boundaries or direct the management of the people for whom the boundary manager is responsible.

"Going around the boss" is common in organizations. It often is done informally, at social occasions, or in other non-discoverable or non-documentable ways; the lack of a written record enables the conveyer of information, if confronted, to deny having done anything wrong.

Example 7
Embarrassing the Manager

A CEO of a large firm was known for embarrassing people in the organization when they failed to deal with a problem in a way, or with the speed, that the CEO desired. In fact, the CEO openly warned individuals, in the midst of staff meetings, that they would be fired if they did not accomplish a particular task or solve a particular problem. Such public pronouncements undermined supervisors' credibility with the employees who reported to them, and those employees tended to distance themselves from the people whom they perceived were losing the CEO's support.

Such situations confuse the boundaries between the functions of CEOs and the functions of the people they supervise. They also violate the boundaries of personal conduct and humiliate the people who are criticized. People who act in this way, at any level, are motivated more by their need to control and dominate than by any conceivable desire to exercise legitimate authority to achieve institutional goals.

One must question the selection processes that enable individuals who violate the boundaries of personal conduct to reach positions of power and influence. In business, such a situation may come about because the CEO, or members of his or her family, founded the business. In other situations, especially in institutions involved in health care, the leader may have been recruited because of his or her technical expertise with little regard to the social boundaries that make for effectiveness in leadership roles.

Example 8
Need for Group Support

A particular division of a medical school department had long been known as a service unit. Its service burdens were so great that few members of the unit ever had been able to write significant grants. While most of them had been promoted and granted tenure, these rewards were given somewhat grudgingly on the basis of their service and teaching support. The two members of the unit who had received funding were the least popular members of the group. In order to find the time to write grants and develop collaborative support, they had shifted some of their service responsibilities to others. Although the division director was aware of the problems created by his "stars," he appreciated the increased regard, on the part of his Chair and the Dean, that their achievements had brought to his division. Discussions with outside staff people helped him realize that to improve morale and productivity, both the psychological and material rewards for the "stars'" achievements had to be shared with the entire unit. Yet, he was faced with a dilemma; the reward system in the medical school seemed to grant power and prestige to "stars" and neglect the other members of the team who make "starring" possible.

In Example 8, the definition of a "good" faculty member is quite different outside and inside of a unit. Outside, service and teaching are taken for granted, and the ability to obtain external funds is highly important. Inside, sharing the workload defines the boundaries. Faculty members who take time off to write grants, or to perform functions related to their grants rather than their service and teaching, are "punished" with unpopularity or resistance. The definition of a "good" faculty member must be enlarged, both inside and outside, so the unit can grow and develop. Narrow definitions of effectiveness, which constitute another type of boundary, produce organizations which neglect a part of their missions. The task of the Division Director and the Chair is to loosen these definitions.

Example 9
The New Broom

The Department of Psychiatry at a medical school had been controlled by an old style of leadership in which a large Private Practice Psychiatry group ran the department. This model, which dominated many American medical schools until after World War II, became obsolete because it did not encourage research or innovation in an era of Federal research funding. Yet, the control of this department by the private group persisted into the 1970's.

After a protacted struggle with the private group and the political support it had acquired, in the 1970's, the Dean hired a charismatic, young psychiatric researcher to Chair the department. The new Chair was advised to break the hold of the private group on the department.

It happened that the most distinguished faculty member in the Department was not a psychiatrist, but a brilliant, internationally known psychologist. This also caused some dissonance in the department; some of the psychiatric faculty believed that psychology had developed an inappropriately strong influence on the psychiatric training of medical students.

The new Chair, taking his role as a "new broom" seriously, not only revoked the faculty appointments of virtually all the members of the private group, but drove all of the psychologists, and most of the psychiatrists, from the Department. For a variety of reasons, relating mostly to the personality of the Chair, many of the Department's new appointees did not stay. As a result, the Department remained in virtual chaos for many years, with little improvement in its research status, although teaching did improve as a result of the modernization of the department's educational program. After about a decade, the Chair left and a new Chair was given the task of improving the department's research and clinical service activities.

In this example, the need for change was evident, but the means were probably unnecessarily painful and disruptive. The Dean and the President had encouraged the Chair's "new broom" approach, but the results may not have been all that they had hoped. The new Chair needed to redefine the boundaries of psychiatry and psychology and also needed to define boundaries that would limit the influence of private practitioners on the Department's activities. It might have been desirable to construct these boundaries in ways that would limit turnover in order to provide for a smooth transition and develop the spirit of collegiality that is essential in maintaining an organization that has a great many service functions. The university lost prestige when the brilliant psychologist left, and the continual personnel changes made it difficult to mount a highly effective research and education program. The Dean recognized the Chair's difficulties with administration, and helped him hire Deputy Chairs who helped rebuild the Department. The whole episode indicates problems with the management of change, and the orientation of change agents. The longer an inappropriate situation exists, the harder it is to make needed changes.

Example 10
The Outsiders

Professional schools require that members of the profession play key roles in administration, but medical education does not prepare physicians for some of the tasks of administration. Physicians generally are not trained for management, education, or community organization. A Dean and his close professional colleague, his Associate Dean, recognized this problem in developing an administrative staff, so they recruited individuals with backgrounds in these fields to staff their Dean's office. While these individuals were talented, there was some grumbling among the clinical department chairs and the senior faculty that the school was being taken over by non-physicians. When a new Dean was appointed, he replaced all three of the non-physician members of his staff, two of them with physicians and the third with a much less proactive administrator.

The replacements, while capable, were somewhat less creative than their predecessors and no more acceptable to the clinical chairs and faculty. The Dean, who is well liked, has been criticized by the faculty for having a relatively mediocre staff.

Organizations in the late twentieth century require a variety of expertise. Boundaries based upon professional snobbery do not contribute the resources necessary for fostering the creativity and imagination necessary for organizational growth and development. Line positions in medical schools, such as Chief Executive Officer and Department Chair, are necessarily filled by physicians or basic medical scientists, but staff positions can be filled by a variety of talented individuals.

Managing Boundaries is Managing People

Organization design theorists, such as Galbraith (1973) and Miller and Rice (1967), argue that boundaries that are poorly designed and managed can cause considerable stress and anxiety. Managers often face the difficult task of finding the right boundary to mark off a work group. A boundary that encompasses too many roles may prove unmanageable, as different role holders pursue different goals and use different tools and resources, e.g., open boundary structure. If a boundary includes too few roles, people inside the boundary may feel unable to influence other role holders on whom they depend, e.g., closed boundary structure (Hirschhorn, 1988). This brings to mind one of Peters and Waterman's (1982) eight basic features of successful companies, i.e., *simultaneous loose-tight properties*, by which they meant that the organizational culture demanded compliance, performance, and obedience to key norms at the same time it permitted an unusual degree of freedom to take risks and innovate.

Fairholm (1991) points out that values dictate organizational action whether they come from individuals or the collective organization. The central task of the manager is to manage value conflicts in favor of a shared value system. Darling and Ogg (1984) stress that common value commitments are key to the interdisciplinary process. The more similarities in values between workers or disciplines, the lower the level of perceived threat, and the greater the likelihood of a team working relationship.

The Value Factor

Managers must be aware that in managing boundaries they are managing value transactions between themselves, employees, and clients, i.e., students and patients. These transactions occur simultaneously on three levels: 1) *internally*, e.g., a person may experience a conflict between valuing honesty on the one hand and the need to protect one's job; 2) *interpersonally*, e.g., managers, the employees, and other groups may rank the same values differently; 3) *culturally*, e.g., those involved in the organization may have different values than those who direct or control the organization. Work values are not inseparable from non-work values. Since most of us spend our lives attempting to satisfy our values or beliefs, it is important to be in touch with people's values continuously if we are to influence or change their behavior.

An example of a value conflict that impedes the effectiveness of both health professions education and health care is the conflict between the so called "academic values" of research oriented faculty and the values of students and patients. Within this larger conflict, there is a tendency to value so called "hard science," e.g., chemistry and physics, and "basic science" compared to "soft science," e.g., psychology and sociology, and "applied science." There is a subtle bias in research funding toward basic research as opposed to applied research. Grants to study basic issues in molecular biology are much easier to fund than grants to investigate the cause of teenage pregnancy or urban violence. This has led to an odd situation in which three of the principal causes of mortality and morbidity in children and young adults—accidents, suicide, and homicide (U.S. Bureau of the Census, 1992)—receive much less funding for study than do much less common or serious problems. Peer review, as admirable as it may be, creates a reluctance to fund studies that reward values different from those of the academicians who form the peer groups. Such biases create second class citizens of health professions faculty who are not basic researchers.

Students are shortchanged by faculty who perceive no rewards in teaching. Academicians interested in investigating clinical care, or developing research in community health, receive much less funding than do those who are interested in the latest preoccupations of the academic community. A vicious circle develops when the most talented individuals are drawn to investigate the "hottest" topics, while other areas, which may be equally important to health care, do not receive funding and are unable to attract talented investigators. This example illustrates how individuals can experience value conflicts arising from their most benevolent impulses. Each side perceives its values to be of paramount importance. Who can say that either basic or clinical research is more important? Some means of assuring that *neither* is neglected needs to be developed.

Dwyer (1981) has acknowledged that values differ significantly among various groups, and that values cannot be debated, since each individual develops values based upon his or her own history and interests. He believes that managers and leaders must seek value rich alternatives so that all the legitimate values and interests in an enterprise can be served. Health professions organizations strive for autonomy, but such autonomy is impossible in today's world. In a democracy, such as the United States, each institution gains power from its ability to convince society that it meets certain social needs. In exchange, society has granted these organizations certain rights and privileges. Managers and leaders, as boundary setters and boundary managers, therefore, have at least three tasks. First, they must advance the values and interests of the larger society, even when their followers do not want to pay attention to greater social needs. At present, deans and presidents of medical schools must reassert the need for attention to primary care in institutions which thrive on tertiary care and attention to teaching in institutions renowned for research. Second, they must try to foresee the changes in boundaries that are bound to occur, and try to protect their institutions from change that is too rapid and destructive. Capricious caps on reimbursements, and support for education and research, can wreak havoc on training institutions and teaching hospitals. Third, they should try to be proactive and creative in developing new and more effective guidelines for patient care and health professions education in a world of cost controls and government mandates regarding education.

Covey (1990) notes that one of the major causes of "people problems" in organizations is unclear, ambiguous, unfulfilled, or conflicting expectations regarding roles and goals. An expectation is a hope, what a person wants from a situation. Each of us comes into a situation with certain implicit expectations based upon our values and beliefs. Covey proposes a performance agreement for avoiding conflicts in expectations and values. There are two pre-conditions to a performance agreement: trust and communication. The agreement should be open and negotiable by either party at any time. The agreement itself should be based on the principle of win/win performance. This approval shifts the focus of management from control to release. Most important, the structure of the organization reinforces the win/win contract as a process of mutual communication and trust.

Hirschhorn (1991) stresses that managing in a team environment gives employees plenty of elbow room to take charge. The manager is the gatekeeper, assuring that the workers are linked to the organizational environment and that the organization's needs are communicated to the workers. Workers manage the work and the manager manages the boundary. Hirschhorn (1991) points out that, in order to be effective, the boundary manager must ensure that workers understand the organization's operating philosophy, must give the workers feedback on their performance, and must negotiate for the resources the workers need to do their work.

The Reflective Manager

Managers are conditioned to approach problems and make decisions on the basis of boundaries. Boundaries become self serving, and problems within and between organizations become chronic, because decisions are limited by boundaries (Schulman, 1976). Schön (1983) has observed that managers live in an organizational system, which may either promote or inhibit reflection-in-action. The culture of an organization also influences the scope and direction of a manager's problem solving. A reflective manager has a "boundaryless" perspective on issues or problems that take in the organization and its environment. This perspective permits experimentation with solutions, which may cross boundaries. Reflective managers experiment with solutions. They do not become immune to new perspectives for solving problems and they involve those who are part of a problem in diagnosing and resolving it.

Managers in the health professions are not known for reflective management. The types of problems that arise between health professions and between health professionals and their patients are fairly prescriptive, as are their solutions. Both the problems and solutions are influenced largely by established boundaries. Lack of trust and communication are factors in the basis of these problems. Solutions that reinforce boundaries help to perpetuate mistrust and poor communication; hence, similar problems recur.

Managers in the health professions often pay little attention to issues other than the management of their internal problems. Frequently, they fail to act on demanding issues that relate to the environment of the health care system until prodded by the government. For example, in the 1970's, most medical schools, prompted by State and Federal mandates and incentives, established departments of family medicine. These departments were expected, by encouraging the development of a new group of primary care physicians, to alleviate the problems that had been created by the fragmentation of the medical profession into groups of subspecialists. Most of the established medical schools in Texas, although they had departments of family medicine, did not require that students take a course in family medicine, thereby failing to take advantage of the educational opportunities afforded by the creation of the new discipline.

The medical school deans recognized the desirability of introducing students to family medicine early in order to encourage them to consider careers in primary care. However, political forces within the schools, which controlled their curricula, managed to stymie any such attempts. Recently, the Texas legislature mandated that all Texas medical schools add courses in family medicine to their junior year curricula.

Intuition and Creativity in Boundary Management

Intuitive managers have been shown to be perceptive of organizational situations and to offer new ways to address problems and opportunities (Harper, 1989). Management can be viewed as a five step process: awareness, understanding, making decisions, initiating change, and achieving desired results. The awareness stage includes identification of where the organization should be in the future as well as where it is now. The understanding stage focuses on mapping the relationships between various factors. During the decision-making stage, the manager processes huge amounts of information. Often the manager does not know which of this information is relevant and which may be incomplete. Managers, therefore, must use their intuition to make decisions about which information to use and how much additional information to gather. When and how to initiate change to achieve the desired result call upon the manager's intuitive skills regarding timing and behavioral expectations.

Intuitive managers are characterized not only by their unique perspectives, but also by their tendency to be perceptive of organizational situations. They find creative ways to address problems and opportunities. Intuitive managers tend to couple intuition with anticipatory management (Harper 1989). They have foresight and insight into possible problems and opportunities.

These characteristics are helpful in managing boundaries because most boundaries are in various stages of change (Agor, 1991). Even relatively fixed boundaries must respond in some degree to external forces and events to maintain their boundary integrity. The creative manager who anticipates the degree and type of change can effectively manage boundary modifications with minimal disruption in the behavior of the people who are affected by the boundary.

Change is a continual process affecting boundaries, yet the rate of change varies. There is always an attempt by organizations, institutions, groups, etc. to modify the effects of change and maintain some semblance of balance or homeostasis (Albrecht, 1987). The key to boundary management is to keep boundaries, which are necessary for maintaining order and direction, from collapsing. The intuitive manager knows the limits of change and the tolerance levels of the people affected by boundary changes. The intuitive manager can prepare people for change and help them to accept it.

Intuition is of importance in "knowing" an individual's or group's values and the degree of importance boundaries have for them in protecting these values. While turf or boundary wars usually are obvious enough so that intuition is unnecessary to diagnose the problem, intuition may be key to resolving the dispute—finding value-rich alternatives. Keeping the warring parties apart is a temporary solution; turf issues will reemerge unless the underlying causes are addressed. Some causes may not be verbalized and the intuition of the manager becomes essential, not only in discovering the causes, but in "trying out" the limits of realignments of roles, boundary responsibilities, or authority (Agor, 1989).

Directed Autonomy

Waterman (1987) stresses that we need to come to grips with the question of management and control versus freedom and empowerment. A balance is needed between freedom and control, a management style that combines the manager's need for control with the employee's need for individuality. If people in an organization know their boundaries, and the manager gets out of the way in protecting these boundaries, some employees may cross boundaries without difficulty. As Waterman (1987) has said, "to get results you loosen the reins" (p. 88) or "give up control to get control" (p. 90). "We are so busy grandstanding with 'crisp decisions' that we don't take time to involve those who have to make the decisions work" (p. 90).

One method of introducing directed autonomy in an organization is "fishbowl management," proposed by Sargent (1978). Fishbowl management puts the manager into close, frequent involvement with superiors, subordinates, and outsiders in organizational objectives and policies. Fishbowl management is a multilevel approach, which motivates employees and managers by increasing the possibility that their ideas will be adopted and implemented and their performance noticed.

Other, more recent techniques of introducing autonomy in the workplace include self-directed work groups, total quality management, total quality service, quality circle teams, linking teams, and horizontal network teams (Denton, 1991).

Autonomy tends to reduce the likelihood of boundary conflicts, especially when three factors are present: 1) all levels of employees are allowed to participate in decision-making; 2) the problem-solving approach is used to resolve problems; and 3) employees are fully involved in goal-setting, decision-making, and open communication across levels. Denton (1991) has described organizations that have attempted to increase autonomy and "flatten the pyramid." A flat horizontal organization is characterized by floating leadership, which is focused around work projects. This type of organization constructs boundaries around the task or project at a given time. Thus, although employees retain their loyalty to the total organization, their loyalty to specific work groups changes as projects change.

Team building is not new, nor is it easy to accomplish (Dyer, 1977). Groups, or teams, are often criticized for wasting time and producing little. Yet, teams and groups can be effective if managers are effective in managing people. Managers too often focus on the task and not on the process. Managers need to manage boundaries, roles, tasks, and the work environment while providing leadership.

Bolman and Deal (1991) have discussed the concept of "reframing." Boundary managers continually reframe change. Boundary fighting and turf wars erupt when managers are wedded to only one or two frames. Restructuring, recruiting, and retraining can be useful levers for change. As Bolman and Deal (1991) have suggested, change is a four dimensional process involving human resources, structural relationships, political alliances, and symbolic attachments. Changing boundaries requires that managers provide clarity, security and realignments so that those affected by change will not lose face. Organizations, such as hospitals, undergo continual change, such as turnover in employees, difficulty in recruiting personnel, and periodic decreases in morale due to long work hours and lack of rewards. To counter such changes, managers must anticipate them and work to realign roles and relationships. Change will result in some conflict and loss for some members of an organization. Change will benefit some members more than others. The challenge is not to try to eliminate change, but to plan and direct it.

Managing Boundaries: From Win/Lose to Win/Win

Substantial changes in how we educate health professionals will be needed if we are to make the delivery of health services more effective, efficient, and humane. Values that stress the importance of credentials and the differential power, prestige, status, and autonomy they give a profession are instilled during the educational preparation of health professionals. Elitism detracts from collaboration and teamwork. Instead of focusing on combining the expertise of different professionals to provide the best care, energy is devoted to protecting one's turf and identity. As a result, students and patients became victims as professionals defend their own interests. More time and energy is expended in making sure the professionals win than in making sure students and patients win. (see Table 7-3).

Much has been said and written about health care teams. The instances in which they work are uncommon throughout much of health care today. As Hirschhorn (1991) points out, in a team environment, empowerment is balanced with collaboration. Team members focus on the task at hand and the team manager manages boundaries. Team teaching and team administered care are based on the premise that a variety of resources can be brought to bear to successfully accomplish a task. However, it is not only bringing resources together, but orchestrating the resources well that makes the combined effort effective. A physician, a nurse, a social worker, and an occupational therapist do not make a team, even if they have a common operating philosophy and task. It is *how* they work together that results in a win/win outcome. The *how* of collaboration can best be learned by modeling, trial and error, and experience.

It is easy to say that we need a behavioral shift in the health professions, a shift from preserving the status quo to behaving in an innovative, cooperative, and aggressive manner. However, behavior changes must be preceded by changes in perceptions and attitudes. The concerned parties—health professionals, their students, and patients—must feel that it is important for all to win, whether it is in regard to quality health education or quality services. A win/lose philosophy has not led to a system of health professions education, or a system of health services delivery, that meets the changing needs of society. Turfism, territoriality, and boundaries have effectively preserved professional interests and benefits. Boundaries between health professionals and patient care have been idealized and protected from all

TABLE 7-3

Perceptions and Boundary Behavior

Perception	Boundary Behavior	Outcome
Boundaries are opportunities for growth	Aggressive, offensive, expansive	Win/win
Boundaries are opportunities to collaborate	Compromising,, innovative, creative, cooperative	Win/win
Boundaries protect and preserve the status quo	Territorial, defensive self-contained	Win/lose

Source: John G. Bruhn

change except that initiated by the health professional. Only recently has the patient been given "rights" and permitted to be an advocate for his/her own care.

Covey (1989) points out that paradigms are inseparable from character. In the human dimension, being is seeing, and what we see is highly interrelated with what we are. Paradigms are powerful because they create the lens through which we see the world. In health professions education and practice, we need to shift from a reactive to a proactive paradigm. We need to develop more flexible boundaries and boundary managers in the health professions.

We need to evolve more participatory, proactive managers who will encourage the development of cross-boundary and interorganizational relationships to address problems and issues. More interaction between disciplines is needed in the education of health professionals if we ever are to have teaming in practice. More problem-based and community-based instruction is needed if future health professions are to understand the impact of other issues on health and the need for committed health professionals to become involved in their total communities. Health

FIGURE 7-2

Development of More Flexible Boundary Managers in Health Organizations

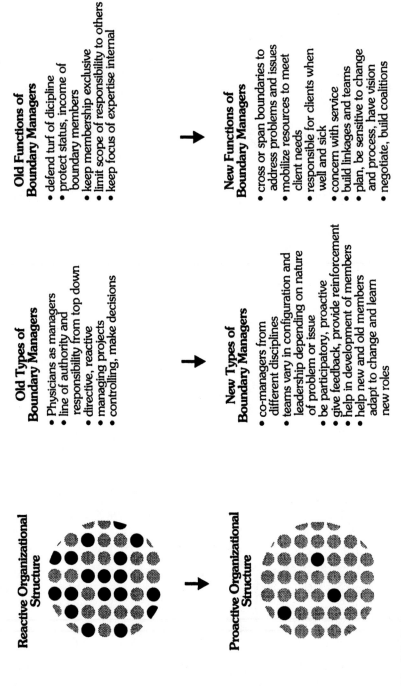

Reactive Organizational Structure

Old Types of Boundary Managers

- Physicians as managers
- line of authority and responsibility from top down
- directive, reactive
- managing projects
- controlling, make decisions

Old Functions of Boundary Managers

- defend turf of dicipline
- protect status, income of boundary members
- keep membership exclusive
- limit scope of responsibility to others
- keep focus of expertise internal

Proactive Organizational Structure

New Types of Boundary Managers

- co-managers from different disciplines
- teams vary in configuration and leadership depending on nature of problem or issue
- be participatory, proactive
- give feedback, provide reinforcement
- help in development of members
- help new and old members adapt to change and learn new roles

New Functions of Boundary Managers

- cross or span boundaries to address problems and issues
- mobilize resources to meet client needs
- responsible for clients when well and sick
- concern with service
- build linkages and teams
- plan, be sensitive to change and process, have vision
- negotiate, build coalitions

Source: John G. Bruhn

professionals will need to loosen their personal and professional boundaries if health services are to truly serve the total person. At present, referral, or sending the patient away, is an easy option. The teaming of professionals, in one location, to serve the patient would seem more convenient, possibly less expensive, and certainly more considerate and responsive to the patient's needs. Health professions should aspire to this value.

Often, all that is required is that one manager take the initiative, discussing how cooperation can be encouraged. Numerous instances in which cross-disciplinary cooperation is needed can be described. Pediatric residents need to learn to do simple sutures. Surgical residents need to develop models for interacting with primary care physicians. Radiology and pathology residents need to learn to be consultants. Physiatrists and orthopedic surgeons need to develop respect for each others' skills and contributions. It is usually because those who are responsible for education in these disciplines feel uncomfortable dealing with equals whose values are different from their own that these needs often go unmet. The potential gains for both trainees and patients are evident. A value structure, which encourages cooperation, and managerial skill in dealing with people and accepting compromises, has been lacking.

Often, lack of cooperation and inappropriate use of resources are rewarded by the system, just as excessive treatment is rewarded by reimbursement systems. Units may receive more rewards in terms of space, income, and flexibility if they maintain closed boundaries. For example, a surgical department that monopolizes all simple surgical techniques may be allocated more residents than it would if pediatric residents were trained to do sutures. In another instance, a medical school department might avoid using such services as biomedical communications because the service departments charge fees. Instead, it may use faculty time to develop posters and design brochures. The fact that such use of faculty time can lead to fewer publications, less teaching activity, and fewer grant awards is seldom recognized. Often, the creative use of management incentives can encourage cooperation and the appropriate use of resources. Surgical departments can receive credit for training pediatric residents, and all departments can receive lump sum allocations that will encourage them to make use of biomedical communications divisions. The sensitivity of management to wasted opportunities for achieving excellence is prerequisite to the exploration of opportunities for cooperation and collaboration.

Healthy Organizations and Healthy Managers

Lyth (1991) has noted that, while challenging, it is possible to change organizations so that they and their members become healthier. While each organization must strive for better health in its own way, the general indices of a healthy organization include: adaptability to change, the ability to plan for and work out problems, the provision of autonomy without undue supervision to personnel, participation by personnel in decision-making, opportunities for people to grow and develop, and managers whose philosophy is guided by principles and values rather than the gratification of their personal needs.

How do organizations become healthier? According to Clark (1969), organizations need to do more than meet the needs of individuals, they also need to consider the needs of individuals to form groups and of the total organization to engage in transactions with other organizations. It is important for individuals and groups within an organization to cross the boundaries drawn by training and skills in order to solve specific problems or produce specific products. Clark refers to this as mobilizing "multi-dimensionally useful behavior," behavior that does not depend upon training, to help solve problems and produce products. An analogy might be drawn between such boundary crossing and the personal participation of passersby in dealing with a car accident on an interstate highway, e.g., stopping bleeding, putting out a fire, pulling a victim from wreckage, calling an ambulance, etc. We seem to put our best team skills to work in emergencies and then revert to separate, carefully guarded worlds of specialism.

We need to put our emergency mind-set to use on a daily basis, teaching health professionals skills to use in a variety of situations, not just preparing them to use specific skills in given situations. These two approaches encourage health professionals to view themselves and their skills in different ways. The former approach encourages students to be flexible and adaptive in applying their skills, while the second approach encourages a more structured way of viewing themselves and their abilities.

If the uniqueness of one's profession and its limits is too thoroughly ingrained and reinforced, it is unlikely that members will be encouraged to cross their professional boundaries or learn about the contributions of other professions. More flexible professional boundaries will encourage exploration, teaming, and respect for the skills of others. It has been said that there are two ways of looking at an idea, inward and outward. An inward perspective encourages a short-term view, usually concerned with protecting boundaries. An outward perspective encourages a long-term view, usually concerned with examining opportunities. Our perspectives in educating health professionals and providing services to clients predominantly have been inward.

Wilber (1981) has noted that to receive an education is to learn where and how to draw boundaries and what to do with the bounded aspects. Boundaries encourage us to look inward or outward, rarely both. Thus, we are encouraged to see people and professions as opposites. The world of opposites is a world of conflict. Every boundary line is a potential battle line. The firmer the boundary lines, the more intense the battles (Wilber, 1981).

We need to develop a win/win philosophy in educating future health professionals. To be more effective in our work, whether it is teaching or treating, we need to become more sensitive to boundaries, their functions and purposes, and we especially need to develop insights into how they might be crossed to provide a better product. This transformation will not occur easily or rapidly; specialists and subspecialist health professionals are not eager to open their boundaries. Innovations in the health professions will come with the evolution of a few brave leaders. As Terman's Law of Innovation states, "If you want a track team to win the high jump you find one person who can jump seven feet, not seven people who can each jump one foot" (Martin, 1973, p. 95).

Frequently, the health professions have depended on medicine to be their pacesetter and have mimicked medicine's academic standards and credentials to establish their creditability with medicine and the public, at the same time, criticizing and attempting to become autonomous from medicine. This pattern of behavior does not encourage innovation or creativity; rather, it encourages the establishment of closed boundaries between health professions. Autonomy from medicine does not ensure that professions will become more effective or successful. It does promote the segmentation of services and the specialization of knowledge, both of which are limited, self-promoting perspectives.

How effective health professionals will be in reexamining and opening boundaries in education and services will depend upon their values. Currently, rather rigid boundaries protect the values of health professionals. The values of clients and patients, on the other hand, are open and exposed as individuals and families attempt to get their health needs met. A reconciliation of the needs of clients and the needs of health professionals is needed. Health obviously is not valued in the same way by clients and professionals. Health will have to be valued differently if health services are to be available, accessible, and affordable to all. Health professionals who teach health professions students will have to see beyond the limits of their professional boundaries and ask, "why am I doing what I am doing—for what purpose?" Their answers will reveal a great deal about the prospects for opening boundaries and for new opportunities in the health professions.

REFERENCES

Agor, Weston H.: *Intuition in Organizations.* New York, Sage, 1989.

Agor, Weston H.: How intuition can be used to enhance creativity in organizations. *The Journal of Creative Behavior, 28:* 11–19, 1991.

Albrecht, Karl: *The Creative Corporation.* Homewood, IL, Dow Jones-Irwin, 1987.

Berne, Eric: *Games People Play.* New York, Grove Press, 1964.

Bolman, Lee G., and Deal, Terrence E.: *Reframing Organizations.* San Francisco, Jossey-Bass, 1991.

Clark, James V.: A Healthy Organization. In Bennis, Warren G., Benne, Kenneth D., and Chin, Robert (eds.): *The Planning of Change.* 2nd ed. New York, Holt, Rinehardt and Winston, 1969.

Covey, Stephen R.: *The 7 Habits of Highly Effective People.* New York, Fireside, 1989.

Covey, Steven R.: *Principle-Centered Leadership.* New York, Summit, 1990.

Darling, Lu Ann, and Ogg, H. Lorraine: Basic requirements for initiating an interdisciplinary process. *Physical Therapy, 64:* 1684–1686, 1984.

Denton, D. Keith: *Horizontal Management.* New York, Lexington, 1991.

Dwyer, Charles F.: *Managing People: Handbook for a Two Day Seminar.* Philadelphia, Wharton School of Business, University of Pennsylvania, 1981.

Dyer, William G.: *Team Building: Issues and Alternatives.* Reading, MA, Addison-Wesley, 1977.

Fairholm, Gilbert W.: *Values Leadership: Toward A New Philosophy of Leadership.* New York, Praeger, 1991.

Galbraith, Jay: *Designing Complex Organizations.* Reading, MA, Addison-Wesley, 1973.

Harper, Stephen C.: Intuition: What separates executives from managers. In Agor, Weston H. (ed.): *Intuition in Organizations.* Newbury Park, CA, Sage, 1989.

Hartmann, Ernest: *Boundaries in the Mind: A New Psychology of Personality.* New York, Basic Books, 1991.

Hirschhorn, Larry: *The Workplace Within: Psychodynamics of Organizational Life.* Cambridge, MA, MIT Press, 1988.

Hirschhorn, Larry: *Managing in the New Team Environment: Skills, Tools, and Methods.* Reading, MA, Addison-Wesley, 1991.

Karasek, Robert, and Theorell, Töres: *Healthy Work.* New York, Basic Books, 1990.

Kast, Fremont Ellis, and Rosenzweig, James E.: *Organization and Management: A Systems and Contingency Approach.* 4th edition. New York, McGraw-Hill, 1985.

Lawrence, W. Gordon (ed.): *Exploring Individual and Organizational Boundaries. A Tavistock Open Systems Approach.* New York, John Wiley, 1979.

Lyth, Isabel Menzies: Changing organizations and individuals: Psychoanalytic insights for improving organizational health. In Kets de Vries, Manford, F.R. and Associates: *Organizations on the Couch.* San Francisco, Jossey-Bass, 1991.

Martin, Thomas L. Jr.: *Malice in Blunderland.* New York, McGraw-Hill, 1973.

Miller, Eric J., and Rice, A. Kenneth: *Systems of Organizations.* London, Tavistock, 1967.

Peters, Thomas, and Waterman, Robert: *In Search of Excellence.* New York, Bantam Books, 1982.

Schneider, Susan C.: Managing boundaries in organizations. In Kets de Vries, Manford, F.R. and Associates: *Organizations on the Couch.* San Francisco, Jossey-Bass, 1991.

Schön, Donald A.: *The Reflective Practitioner.* New York, Basic Books, 1983.

Schulman, Paul R.: The reflexive organization: On decisions, boundaries and the policy process. *The Journal of Politics, 38:* 1014–1023, 1976.

Sargent, Howard: *Fishbowl Management.* New York, Wiley, 1978.

Stevens, George H.: *The Strategic Health Care Manager.* San Francisco, Jossey-Bass, 1991.

Sturgess, Gary L.: *Why do good fences make good neighbors? Trends in public sector management.* Paper presented at a meeting of the Royal Australian Institute of Public Administration, New South Wales Division, Sydney, Australia, July 3, 1991.

U.S. Bureau of the Census. *Statistical Abstract of the United States: 1992.* 112th edition. Washington, U.S. Bureau of the Census, 1992.

Vaughn, Donna G. and Bamberg, Richard: *Hospital Utilization of Multiskilled Health Practitioners: A National Perspective.* Birmingham, AL, School of Health Related Professions, University of Alabama, May, 1989.

Waterman, Robert: *The Renewal Factor.* New York, Bantam, 1987.

Wilber, Ken: *No Boundary.* Boston, New Science Library, 1981.

SUMMARY

This book is about social and psychological boundaries and how they affect the performance and behavior of health professionals. It is designed to increase the reader's awareness of the existence of boundaries, the effects of boundaries, and the ways in which knowing about and understanding boundaries can help one cope with their influence.

Boundaries are necessary. They help focus responsibility and mitigate confusion in the performance of one's occupational role. Inappropriate boundaries, however, can stifle initiative, damage morale, cause nonfunctional conflict, and, therefore, damage the efficiency and effectiveness of the people they affect.

We begin by discussing the origin of boundaries, which are rooted in evolution. All living creatures exhibit some territorial behavior and, therefore, must have boundaries to demarcate their territories from those of others. Territories and hierarchies minimize conflict and provide a sense of security and place.

Social and psychological boundaries exist in our minds; they are a function of our perceptions and personalities. We construct these boundaries in order to make our world more predictable and controllable. Some boundaries are constructed to group people who have similar characteristics, behavior, and goals. Such groupings help us feel comfortable and secure. Other boundaries are constructed to protect our economic, social, and professional territories from intrusion.

We describe various boundaries that have arisen among the health professions in America, and discuss how factors, such as elitism, sexism, racism, economic conflicts, etc., have influenced them. While burgeoning technology has led to dramatic decreases in morbidity and mortality in the American population, costs have grown greatly, and some individuals, the poorest and most disadvantaged among us, have difficulty accessing the health care system. Boundary issues and conflicts, which have raised costs and limited access, can threaten the future progress of the system.

We discuss the impact of the personalities and values of health professionals, and of leaders and managers of health profession's schools and institutions, on the management of boundaries. Individual health professionals have learned to be competitive, have survived tough competition to gain entrance into and graduate from their professional schools. Health professionals jealously guard their uniqueness and the status they believe they have earned. As the health field grows more specialized, more unique territories, which need to be guarded, are created.

Unfortunately, patients can become enmeshed in boundary conflicts. As professionals become specialists, and restrict their territories, or expertise, patients find that no one is looking at their problems as a whole. They have become sick lungs, malfunctioning livers, and recalcitrant kidneys. In such a context, physical causes that cut across organ systems are neglected, and psychosocial problems are ignored.

A few boundary spanners do exist in the health professions, primary care professionals who tend to view problems in their holistic context. Examples of such boundary spanners are the family physician, the nurse practitioner, the physician's assistant.

We have pointed out several examples of boundary conflicts between groups of health professionals and speculated on their effects on the quality of patient care. Some boundary conflicts are due, not to the direct intervention of people, but to the effects of the products they produce. Technology, which has clear and obvious benefits, also has negative effects that often are less obvious. New technologies require new skills, which usually result in the creation of new disciplines and, consequently, new boundaries. Increased boundaries, and the complex interplay between subspecialties, make the attempt to create teams, and to deliver comprehensive services that have continuity to clients, a managerial nightmare.

People who attempt to cross boundaries are not only brave; if they are to be successful, they must exert strong leadership. At the organizational level, leaders who wish to manage boundaries have to define a mission and protect its integrity. At the individual level, leaders must manage the complex relations between themselves and their followers. Boundary issues involve the personalities, values, and beliefs of the manager and the managed. For example, some managers may feel a need to dominate and control, which will predispose them to rigid boundaries. Others may have a more laissez faire approach, and their boundaries will be more porous. They may believe that employees are basically untrustworthy, which would result in different boundaries than would thinking most people are to be trusted. They may value client services, or profit making effectiveness, adherence to tradition, or humane treatment of employees. All of these values influence the types of boundaries that are established.

Trust is the lubrication that allows organizations to work and employees to grow professionally. Managers who do not trust, or who create an environment of continual change and turnover, cultivate a climate of fear, of striving to protect one's job, and a lack of organizational loyalty. In such an organizational climate, boundaries are constantly in flux so that employees do not know how to perform their jobs. In the health professions, we need to develop managers who will provide a secure enough setting to allow employees to span boundaries to provide effective services to patients.

Boundaries in organizations can be described in different ways with respect to their permeability, focus, and changeability. Boundaries must be strong enough to maintain responsible behavior within organizations, but permeable enough to allow cooperation between discrete organizations working toward a common goal. The stability of an organization's boundaries is determined largely by the boundary manager. The job of a manager is to shift boundaries, both inside and out, so that others can work effectively, anticipating boundary problems and mitigating them.

In addition to the technological changes that we have mentioned, social, cultural, economical, and political changes have resulted in such long standing conflicts as those between medicine and pharmacy, dentistry and dental auxiliaries, occupational therapy and physical medicine. We discuss ways in which such conflicts can be alleviated.

We discuss ways in which organizations can alleviate the stresses of boundary change and develop methods of bridging boundaries and developing effective health care teams. We have provided some actual examples of boundary conflicts and an opportunity for readers to try to analyze some difficult conflicts in terms of boundary management.

This book has used the health professions as a backdrop for discussing the concept of boundaries and their dynamics. Health professions are not the only groups or organizations that encounter or experience boundary conflicts, change, and instability. Most of what we have discussed also applies to the non-health world, indeed, to the management games of daily life. Hopefully, we have provided some insights and guidelines to encourage the improvement of boundary management. Each reader could multiply our examples tenfold. It is the process of reflection and study about boundaries that we hope to promote and encourage.

APPENDIX A

Guidelines For Managing Boundaries

The following general guidelines are offered to help managers recognize and analyze boundaries. In doing so, they may be able to prevent boundary wars and maintain and direct the productive functions of boundaries in organizations and groups. Note that employees are not the only ones affected by boundaries. Patients are put at risk when different specialists do not collaborate effectively for their optimal care, and trainees (students, residents, and fellows) are affected by institutional boundaries.

I. Awareness of Boundaries

Managers first must increase their awareness of boundaries. Sometimes, a manager is unaware of the significance of boundaries until a "turf war" erupts. Boundaries exist whether or not we see them. They usually perform a valuable function in a group or organization. However, boundaries that are not managed can be disruptive and destructive.

II. Know Boundary Types

Second, it is important to learn about and reflect upon the different types of boundaries and their locations within an organization. The larger the organization, the greater the variety of boundaries, and, therefore, the greater the complexity of their interactions. Knowing the types of boundaries they are dealing with, permits managers to "stand back," observe the subtleties of interaction between people, and gain insights into current or future problems.

III. Know Boundary Members

Belonging to a group or organization has different meanings for different people. The more important a group, and what it represents to its members, the greater the intensity with which its members will defend the group. We all obtain satisfaction from membership in groups. Because this satisfaction is important to them, people become mobilized to act when their boundaries are threatened. Managers must be aware of the importance of a group's boundaries to its members and its clients if they are to understand the strength of the feelings engendered by boundaries.

229

IV. Consider Boundary Options

Managers should be flexible and consider a variety of options when boundary changes are planned. The options considered by management may not be the same options perceived by members. Dialogue between boundary representatives and management, regarding change, its effects, trade-offs, and future implications, is essential.

V. Awareness of Boundary Interactions

Boundaries exist in systems of varying complexity. All boundaries, of all types, are affected by the environment in which they exist. Managers cannot control or comprehend all of the obvious and subtle effects that influence the behavior of members and clients of their group or organization. Yet, managers must be aware of the effect of boundary changes on other parts of the organization.

VI. Prevent Boundary Wars

Most boundary wars can be prevented. Managers must be aware of the signs and symptoms preceding "boundary tiffs," before they escalate. Boundary wars usually occur because those affected by the boundaries have been unable to gain the attention of managers and feel helpless to change their situations. The most extreme type of boundary war is a strike or walk-out. More moderate types include work slowdowns, absenteeism, thefts, etc. Sometimes, the groups excluded or disadvantaged by boundaries appeal to the political process, e.g., try to change licensure acts, or the legal process, e.g., file antitrust suits. It is tempting for managers to assume that discontent is the fault of a few individuals without delving more deeply into the reasons. Therefore, they often delay giving boundary skirmishes their attention until they become full blown boundary wars.

VII. Build Trust and Communication

Some groups become closed because they do not trust others. Where there is a lack of trust, there is, undoubtedly, a lack of communication. If managers and personnel do not talk with each other, distrust is bound to follow. As a result, the barriers between management and boundary groups become firmly established and protected. Managers must be good listeners regarding the needs and interests of trainees, clients, and employees. Those groups may establish boundaries to protect their needs. If groups suffering from boundary problems believe that an organization is open about meeting their needs, they will be less defensive. Trust is established by a track record. Organizations and managers must prove themselves to be open and receptive if they expect openness and receptivity from their clients and employees.

VIII. Know Your Management Style

Managers must know themselves well to manage others. Numerous personality and other inventories allow people to test their personality dimensions and learn about themselves. Managers may find them helpful. Managers manage by exhibiting their values. How managers treat other people, especially, how they manage conflict and change, tells a lot about their value systems. Managers have personal boundaries and belong to a variety of groups with varying boundary structures. The groups that managers belong to reflect their values. Managers must be aware of their biases, experiences, and values as they address boundary issues that impinge on their organizations.

APPENDIX B

Vignettes for Discussion

Following are a number of vignettes drawn from a wide variety of situations involving the health professions and health professionals. In reviewing each vignette, consider the following questions:

- What boundary issues does this vignette present?
- What can be done to resolve the present conflict between individuals and groups?
- What past behaviors might have prevented the present problems?

Vignette #1
"Precious Space"

Two Schools shared a new, multi-million dollar building on a health science center campus. During its construction, the two deans and their faculties had input into the space arrangements in the building and delineated which space would be shared and which utilized by only one school. School B had a larger faculty and a need for more laboratories; hence, School B was given a larger share of the building. Shortly after the building was completed, the Dean of School A left. The new dean was aggressive in seeking grants and expanding programs. School B was less aggressive and, therefore, less successful in obtaining outside funding. The Dean of School A soon ran out of space for added personnel and, therefore, asked the Dean of School B to relinquish some space to School A, which he did. This required some renovation, which disrupted sections of the building in which faculty of the two schools were housed. Faculty members of School B became quite vocal in their criticism of School A and its expansion. The Dean of School B could not justify to the Vice President for Academic Affairs the use of faculty offices in his area for departmental libraries, storage, or coffee rooms. The relinquishment of space to School A was resented by the faculty of School B, even after given the rationale for giving up the space. The faculty of School B perceived that School A was "taking over the building," despite the fact that ample space for School B remained even after some was given up.

Both Deans, with some faculty pressure, approached the President with a plan to add two additional floors to the five year old building, one floor to accomodate the projected expansion of each school. Although the original justification for the new building was the practicality of teaching space that could be shared, the person who scheduled rooms found competition for the same rooms in the new building keen among faculty from both schools. Some faculty members booked rooms a year in advance, or booked several rooms for the same class until they knew their class size. Ironically, some seminar rooms in the building were never used.

The clashes between faculty and staff, usually over minor, easily resolved issues, were frequently brought to the attention of the Deans. Resentment among the building's occupants was constant, as was the feeling that one of the two schools should not be there.

Vignette #2
"Toppling the Leader"

A department in a health professions school in a university had been working toward accreditation for several years. Several department chairs had come and gone because they did not believe the university administration was supporting their program and because the department's faculty was divisive and subject to frequent turn-over.

Advertisements for a new departmental chair did not yield an acceptable candidate. One faculty member applied for the position, but was not interviewed. Instead, the Dean appointed, as ad interim chair, a health professional who was directing a graduate level program in the discipline that was being extended from the university's mother campus. The faculty members in the department were in the midst of preparing materials for accreditation. They were incensed that an outside candidate who had been interviewed was not hired and that none of them had been considered for the interim chair position. Some of the faculty members mobilized the students against the administration. The students asked for a meeting with administrative representatives. The meeting was confrontational and hostile; the students presenting prepared questions for which they wanted answers. The administrative representatives reaffirmed their support for the program as evidenced by a search for a director, payment of the appropriate fees for accreditation, and the purchase of additional library books and journals in the discipline. The administration surmised that the faculty candidate who wanted to be chair, but was not interviewed, was instrumental in mobilizing the students and assisting them with their questions.

The appointed interim chair resigned when it became apparent that four faculty members were united against him. The Dean then asked the four faculty members to name an interim chair from among themselves while the search for a permanent chair was conducted. Meanwhile, the students wrote a letter of complaint to the accrediting agency, thereby jeopardizing the accreditation of their program.

Vignette #3
"New Beginnings"

Downsizing (also known as rightsizing) in an organization causes the establishment of new boundaries. Consolidation and reorganization, which result in the lay-off of workers, a reexamination of the goals and functions of a unit, and a reorientation of management, all can cause a great deal of uncertainty, fear, and anger among workers. On the other hand, downsizing can result in a more cohesive and efficient organization, forcing remaining employees to function as a team to accomplish necessary tasks.

A large health science center more sharply focused its mission as a result of severe budget deficits. The President and several ad hoc faculty advisory committees decided that, in the future, the center would support only graduate degree programs. All baccalaureate programs, not crucial to the mission of the center, would be closed or transferred to other clinical facilities or departments.

It was interesting to see how cooperative departments were in this reorganization. Departments, which previously balked at providing financial support for baccalaureate programs, offered space, faculty, and equipment to continue the programs under their auspices. Hospitals, which, earlier, had offered sign-on bonuses to attract baccalaureate health professionals in short supply, formed coalitions with other hospitals to support a program which was faced with closure. A nearby university, which had competed with the health science center for applicants to some baccalaureate programs, offered to expand their programs to accommodate more students if the health science center would, in turn, accept their students in a variety of clinical internships.

While these new arrangements did not necessarily result in cost savings, they did ensure the continuation of programs in which a variety of health providers had an interest. Competition evolved into cooperation. Boundaries, which, formerly, separated the health science center from local hospitals, and separated departments within the health science center, were erased. Obviously, new boundaries will be established as these programs assume new identities.

Vignette #4
"Grieving for Attention"

The fifteen some employees in a work unit complained to the university's EEO Officer that their manager was increasingly intolerable. The manager was characterized as demanding, verbally abusive, insensitive to ethnic minorities, and unwilling to listen. Employee turnover had increased, yet the administrative head of the unit supported the manager, calling him competent and effective. The EEO Officer presented the administrative head with the employee's complaints, and counseled him regarding rectifying the situation. The administrative head, in turn, met with the manager to discuss the complaints. The administrative head was optimistic that the manager would change his behavior. A few weeks later, however, the manager said he intended to file a grievance against his employees for uncooperative and complaining behavior. The administrative head than saw a different side of his manager, stating, "he doesn't listen." The grievance process had become a weapon for the manager and his employees to use against each other, requiring that the university vice president intercede in the face of the declining morale of this work unit. The vice president counseled with the administrative head about ways to cope with the decline in morale, turnover in staff, and the increased critical comments by the employees to others on the university campus.

Vignette #5
"Dominance by Another Profession"

Some time ago, one of the medical specialties decided that it would be helpful if a group of technical level personnel could be trained to perform some of the specialists' laboratory functions. Since complex procedures were required, and the medical specialists would be unable to supervise every procedure, the technologists in question would have to be competent to take responsibility for their work. Therefore, a position was created that would require baccalaureate degree candidates, after three years of college, to spend one year in a hospital laboratory mastering the technical procedures. The medical specialty provided quasi-licensure for the new professionals, granting them certification once they passed a qualifying examination and signed an agreement that they would work only for physicians. Should any of the new technologists work in facilities managed by non-physician scientists, they would lose their certification.

The number of new professionals grew, and the profession became organized. The certification examination committee was expanded to include members of the new profession. Nevertheless, the new professionals resented the restrictions on the content of their certifying examination, the requirements for their professional schools, and the requirements for their employability that were imposed by the medical specialists.

The passage of Medicare greatly expanded the value of the technologists' certificate since Federal guidelines required certification of employees in facilities that accepted Medicare money. Complaints to the Federal government modified the control of the new professionals' professional schools, and an anti-trust suit by the Federal government eliminated the threat of loss of certification. However, resentment and anger have persisted between the two professional groups. The technical level group established its own certification procedures, thereby giving its members two paths to certification.

Vignette #6
"Conflict Among Specialists"

The guidelines for accreditation of pediatric residency programs require that pediatric residents receive some experience in a particular surgical specialty. One pediatric residency program, for a time, required that each resident spend a month on that surgical service during his/her third year of training. For several years, the pediatric residents complained that the surgeons did not seek their advice, and that the rotation was a waste of time. The Department of Pediatrics terminated the rotation. Its residency program is now out of compliance with the requirements of the Residency Review Committee in Pediatrics.

Vignette #7
"Chiropractic"

Chiropractic, as a profession, developed independently of allopathic medicine. For many years, the American Medical Association labeled chiropractic, "quackery," and, until restrained by a Federal Department of Justice anti-trust suit, tried, by various means, to destroy the chiropractic profession. At the present time, many patients visit both types of professionals. In fact, even allopathic physicians sometimes visit chiropractors for treatment of certain ailments. However, the two healing professions have no official contact with each other.

Vignette #8
"Training in Data Gathering"

Two fundamental skills required of all physicians are the taking of patient histories and the conducting of physical examinations. Medical students, however, are rarely observed performing either activity. In one medical school, a freshman course has been designed to teach these skills. The recruitment of clinicians to teach this course is so difficult that many of the small groups' leaders, who are supposed to teach medical interviewing, are basic scientists who have no experience in such interviewing. The physical examination part of the course is taught by volunteer senior medical students who, themselves, may be inadequate. Thus, one of the most important tasks of clinical medical education is neglected by the clinical faculty.

Vignette #9
"A Loose Cannon"

A faculty member in a large university was well known for his outbursts of temper and for his complaining memos to the higher administration, including the President, when things did not go his way. No person in the university was exempt from his periodic wrath. When he perceived that the administration was too slow in getting a new graduate degree approved for his department, he organized a student sit-in in the Office of the Vice President for Academic Affairs. Indeed, he admitted students to the program before it was approved. When he and a group of 40 students and faculty from his department confronted the Vice President, the faculty member announced that he had come to "kick ass."

This faculty member was extremely productive in scholarly activities, and brought in many funded grants. He was known as a dedicated teacher and a genius in his field. Because of his positive contributions to the university, his temper tantrums and memos were tolerated. Administrators and other faculty members walked on egg shells to avoid irritating him. It was never known when this faculty member might go into a tirade or who would be his next target.

Vignette #10
"Lobbying for Promotion and Tenure"

Each year, the Department, College, and Dean of a medium-sized university review faculty applications for promotion and tenure and make recommendations to the Vice President for Academic Affairs. The Vice President then reviews the materials and submits recommendations to the President of the University. The President makes the final decision. The process is well known on campus. Attempts are made to keep the process fair, as unbiased as possible, and timely. Because of the various steps in this process, several months elapse before the outcome is known to the faculty.

A faculty member in a College, whose family was a large donor to the University and a friend of the President, was in her penultimate year for consideration for tenure. The Department voted for granting tenure, but both the College and the Dean recommended against it. Before the Vice President reviewed her file, he received phone calls and letters from faculty members and a request for an appointment from the faculty applicant. There was concern that faculty applicants were being judged by the new College Dean's new guidelines for promotion and tenure, which were more stringent than those that had been in use, even though they were not yet in effect—they had not been voted on by the college faculty.

Some faculty members of the Department and College, who were friends of the faculty applicant, began to lobby on her behalf. Faculty in the Department began to criticize the Dean for not having the new guidelines in place. Faculty members who had recently joined the College were "confused and angry" about which set of standards would be applied to them. One or two outspoken faculty members talked about a law suit if the applicant under review was not given tenure. Under the "old" guidelines, this applicant was considered tenurable.

The Vice President declined to meet with faculty members or the applicant, or to respond to letters from faculty members, until he had reviewed the file. He did, however, confer with the College's Dean.

INDEX

239

J

Japan
    management traits in, 112
    work roles in, 65
Japanese, 13
Jews, 13, 15, 17, 44
Job discrimination
    protection against, 6:16
    sex-related, 5:32
Job involvement, 4:32
Job responsibilities, boundaries of, 139
Job satisfaction, 59, 60, 61, 65, 123, 178
    boundary spanning activity, correlation
        with, 57
    factors in determining, 60
Job titles and descriptions, references to sex
        and age, elimination of, 169
Joint ventures, 31, 148

K

Koop, C. Everett, 105

L

Labeling, 8, 25–28
Labels, 112
    indicators of boundaries, as, 26
    pre-labels, 27
Labor and delivery, 16
Lakeshore Mental Health Institute, Memphis,
    179
Language barriers, 29
Latins, 13
Lawyers, female, 154, 170
Leader-follower relationship, 106, 117
Leadership, 105, 106–110, 128, 226
    behavior, 117, 125
        democratic or participative, 117
        directive, 4:21
        supportive, 4:36
    definition, 4:4
    employee centered, 4:22
    floating, 215
    formal, need for, 178, 179
    management, difference from, 146
    models, 177
    practices, 117

production centered, 117
research, 106
roles, effectiveness in, 206
skills, 117
styles, 106–108, 117, 196, table 197
    styles of managing, relationships with,
        196
task-oriented, 106
tasks, 106–108, 128
theories, 106
Leadership model, Tannenbaum-Schmidt, 177
Licensed Practical Nurse (LPN), 85
Licensure, 19, 20, 40, 134
    examinations, 19
    professional, 19
    state, 40
Lincoln, Abraham, 105
Locus of control, 127
Long-term care, 97

M

Magnetic resonance imaging (MRI), 148
Male work groups, resistance to females of,
    154
Management
    anticipatory, 213
    control, 180
    fishbowl, 214
    incentives, creative use of, 219
    participative, 182, 185
    problems associated with boundary
        structures, table 126
    reflective, 212
    traits in, Japanese and American, 113
Management style(s), 58, 106, 110–113,
        117–119, table 126, 181–182, 190,
        196–202, 231
    components of, 111
    employee adaption to, 113
    leadership, difference from, 146
    leadership, relationship with, 196
    victims of, 113
Managerial
    control system, 58
    flexibility, strategic, 115
    problem solving, 212
Managers
    accessibility to employees, 110